Wheat Syndromes

Detlef Schuppan • Kristin Gisbert-Schuppan

Wheat Syndromes

How Wheat, Gluten and ATI Cause Inflammation, IBS and Autoimmune Diseases

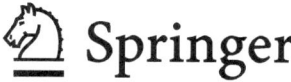 Springer

Detlef Schuppan
Institute of Translational Immunology
University Medical Center
Mainz
Germany

Division of Gastroenterology
Beth Israel Medical Center
Harvard Medical School
Boston, MA
USA

Kristin Gisbert-Schuppan
Institute of Translational Immunology
University Medical Center
Mainz
Germany

ISBN 978-3-030-19022-4   ISBN 978-3-030-19023-1   (eBook)
https://doi.org/10.1007/978-3-030-19023-1

This Springer imprint is published by the registered company Springer Nature Switzerland AG
The registered company address is: Gewerbestrasse 11, 6330 Cham, Switzerland

Preface

This book is different from any other book on wheat, gluten, and nutrition because it is a profoundly medical book. Although it is a profoundly medical book, not one of the many a-little-bit-medical but otherwise popular guidebooks on lifestyle, diet, or cooking, we can assure you that it won't be dry or boring. On the contrary, we would like to take you on for a thrilling journey of discovery and insight, a scientific and clinical expedition to which we have dedicated decades of our lives as researchers and clinicians. When we took off on our exploration, well equipped with a reasonable armamentarium and curiosity, we didn't know what we were going to find, and it is still surprising for us which previously unknown realms we had entered and got to know. We would like you to join us on this journey and invite patients, doctors, and everybody interested alike.

What we have found is completely different from anything you have ever heard about in the fields of nutrition or medicine. We are all used to the observation that people tolerate different foods better or worse, but our food does normally not cause serious harm (apart from common allergies) or make people seriously ill when consumed in moderate amounts. This is what distinguishes food from the inedible. You might reply: But some authors and books claim exactly this—that foods can be poisonous, especially wheat and gluten. We would answer back: Where is their scientific and mechanistic evidence? Where are their scholarly papers? Have these authors got involved in the hardships of scientific expeditions and clinical studies? We would be open to learning about their evidence—we cannot see it. If our insights were not really new and different, we would not have written this book.

Our journey consists precisely of this scientific adventure that others have not bothered to embark on. We have accomplished this expedition through scientific research and extensive clinical care for patients in major university hospitals, namely, at the Beth Israel Deaconess Medical Center of Harvard Medical School, Boston, MA, and at our Research Institute for Translational Immunology at the University Medical Center in Mainz, Germany. What is protocolled in the logbook of our explorations has been published in high-ranking scientific journals in which only papers are accepted that expert colleagues classify as novel, relevant, and scientifically outstanding. We will present theses scientific results to you in digestible and appetizing portions in the following chapters. In addition to the scientific logbook, we brought home our clinical logbook, so to speak, in which the in-depth work with our patients in the United States and in Germany is reflected. All too often, our patients are highly complicated cases that came from year-long odysseys through the medical system, where they had not found the clinical information and professional understanding that they needed. How we were able to help these patients and how the results of our research endeavors helped us to do so are what we are presenting our readers in the following chapters.

What are the unknown territories that we have charted so far? Our discoveries go far beyond what was known in nutrition and nutritional medicine. When we started, there was an exception to the well-known rule that a staple food consumed in moderation cannot cause illness, and this exception is also related to wheat: *celiac disease*. In 1997, we discovered the *celiac disease autoantigen*, published in the journal *Nature Medicine*, and thus laid the foundation to finally understand the mechanism why a common foodstuff, gluten, causes serious symptoms in celiac patients. With this discovery, we also established the urgently needed safe blood test that allowed to screen populations and detect this severe hidden disease that had been responsible for a widespread failure to thrive in infants and misery in children and adults. Because gluten is the culprit of celiac disease, many people believe or are made to believe that gluten can also be harmful to non-celiacs. This is grossly wrong, as you will learn in this book. Apart from its historical paradigm-changing role in medicine, we present celiac disease in our book in much detail, because it is still not well understood by practitioners, severely underdiagnosed in patients, and one of the most important differential diagnoses of the novel diseases we describe in the following chapters.

In this book, we present for the first time to a public outside the scientific community two novel diseases caused by defined components of wheat, other than gluten. One disease is *atypical wheat allergy* (there are also *classical wheat allergies* that are rare and have been known for some time). *Atypical allergies* are a brand new but already well-defined disease entity that was discovered by us along with our London-based friend and colleague Annette Fritscher-Ravens[1]. *Atypical wheat allergy* will be a common diagnosis in the near future. It affects predominantly the intestine and leads almost exclusively to symptoms there. Because nothing like this was known before, it has not been recognized as a form of allergy, and persons affected are usually classified as patients with "irritable bowel syndrome" (IBS), a diagnosis that, due to our discovery, will largely vanish. Besides wheat, there are other atypical allergies. Prominent are milk, soy, and yeast. Since symptoms are delayed, most patients cannot associate allergen consumption with their complaints. Our patients, in whom we have diagnosed atypical allergies with a special procedure, have all become symptom-free under the allergen-free diet. Since 10–15% of most populations worldwide have an atypical food allergy, about 60% to wheat, all healthcare systems in the world will have to realize the real cause of "IBS" because

---

[1] See Chap. 7.

today, it leads to immense, unnecessary costs and human suffering that can easily be avoided.

The other hitherto unknown territory that we were the first to enter on our research journey turned out to be a true continent: the continent of ATI (amylase trypsin inhibitors). Scientifically and clinically, our findings brought about a highly relevant paradigm change in the field of immunology. Our results will also change how people look at the staple food no. 1 worldwide: wheat. With the ATI, we have been able to decipher the importance of a certain class of proteins in wheat—with extremely surprising results for human health. ATI interfere with every attack and defense maneuver within the human body, making unexplainable symptoms and phenomena understandable for the first time.

However, what do ATI do? The ATI that we consume with our daily bread and wheat-based meals activate the stems and branches of innate and adaptive immunity. What these complicated mechanisms of innate and adaptive immunity mean and how they are to be understood, we will guide you through. We will show you the way through the fascinating terrain of the gut's immunology and its interaction with the entire body. What should be known already at this point: ATI heat up and worsen all diseases in which inflammatory processes play a role. We present hard data to you, showing that ATI adversely affect different classes of diseases. One class is autoimmune diseases, such as inflammatory bowel diseases, multiple sclerosis, rheumatoid arthritis, scleroderma, or lupus. Autoimmune diseases are widespread; according to the AARDA,[2] approximately 50 million Americans, 20% of the population are affected. Other diseases that are promoted by ATI are the many forms of life-threatening progressive fibrotic diseases (e.g., lung, liver, and kidney fibrosis), as well as the prevalent and grossly underestimated chronic fatigue syndrome, and even several forms of cancer. ATI are also decisive drivers of all the so-called civilization diseases that the western world and increasingly the whole world have to struggle with. Thus, we have proof that ATI contribute to obesity, metabolic syndrome, fatty liver, NASH, and type 2 diabetes. With the discovery of ATI and the understanding of the mechanisms of how they work in the human body, we have identified a vicious nutrient. If we succeed in eliminating ATI, we will have an enormous impact on world health.

Taken together, this book is about how we set foot in the newly discovered country of atypical allergies as well as the newly discovered whole continent of ATI that nobody had known about before. Join us on our journey. We can promise that you will get a completely new view of the world of nutrition and health.

Mainz, Germany   Detlef Schuppan
July 2019   Kristin Gisbert-Schuppan

---

[2] American Autoimmune Related Diseases Association, Inc. (https://www.aarda.org/)

Acknowledgments by Detlef Schuppan

First, I thank all my patients whom I have seen over decades in Boston, MA, and in Mainz, Germany, and who have trusted and supported me in my explorations and scientific work, knowingly and unknowingly. Without their openness and trust, the progress that is documented in this book would not have been possible.

I am also deeply grateful to my colleagues and co-workers both in the United States and in Germany: graduate, PhD, and MD students, postdoctoral fellows, and national and international collaborators. They have been keys to a diverse, lively, and fertilizing lab, research, and clinical community, without whom, the discoveries, research, and clinical studies that are presented in this book would not have been possible. The creative synergy of these diverse contributors from more than 20 nations continues to be a fruitful ground for novel discoveries and progress. Their names are engraved in the many joint publications on wheat and food sensitivities.

I am particularly indebted to my valued colleague Prof. Annette Fritscher-Ravens, MD, who first discovered real-time food reactions in the small intestine and became my closest collaborator in the field of atypical food allergies.

We have written this book for our children, Darwin, Suldano, Renana, and Sahra, who always follow our endeavors with deep interest and tolerated our preoccupation with this work.

My greatest thanks go to my wife and coauthor, Kristin Gisbert-Schuppan, PhD. Every single part of this book is the result of our joint effort. For me, her view as a clinical psychologist, psychoanalyst, and experienced author was crucial to delve into the creative process that led to this unique book that equally addresses medical experts as well as patients. But apart from working together on this book, Kristin is an indispensable part of my entire work—as of my whole life.

Contents

About the Authors

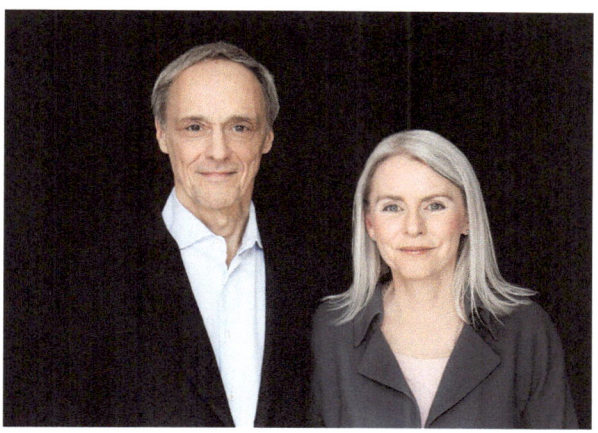

Detlef Schuppan, MD, PhD, is director of the Institute of Translational Immunology at Mainz University Medical Center in Germany. He is also Professor of Medicine in the Division of Gastroenterology at the Beth Israel Deaconess Medical Center and Harvard Medical School in Boston, MA, USA. He made major contributions in the fields of intestinal and liver diseases, examples of which include the identification of the autoantigen of celiac disease, tissue transglutaminase; discovery of wheat amylase-trypsin inhibitors as triggers of ATI sensitivity; the new entity of atypical food allergies as a major cause of irritable bowel syndrome (IBS); key works in the diagnosis and treatment of fibrotic diseases, especially liver fibrosis and cirrhosis, to name a few. He runs a lab with numerous well-funded research projects and worldwide collaborations. His outpatient clinic is unique and currently focuses on patients with complicated and often undiagnosed food-related, intestinal, autoimmune, and liver diseases.

Kristin Gisbert-Schuppan, PhD, is a clinical psychologist, psychotherapist, and psychoanalyst. She works in private practice and at the Institute of Translational Immunology at Mainz University Medical Center in Germany. Her research focuses on narrative and psychosomatic aspects of food-related and autoimmune diseases.

Chapter 1
Introduction

The core part of this book comprises three comprehensive clinical chapters (Chaps. 4, 5, and 7) and two basic chapters (Chaps. 2 and 3). Chapter 2 provides a brief overview of the history of wheat cultivation and breeding, and of the major wheat proteins that play a causative role in the wheat sensitivities. Chapter 3 explains the anatomy of the intestine and provides an easy-to-understand description of the complex intestinal immune system, whose task is to identify food components as friend or foe. The clinical chapters broadly cover the 3 wheat sensitivities: 1. celiac disease, 2. wheat (and other food) allergies, especially the newly discovered atypical allergies, and 3. ATI sensitivity (ATI = amylase trypsin inhibitors). All three diseases cause inflammation and must, therefore, be taken seriously.

ATI-sensitivity, the centerpiece of our book (Chap. 5), is a completely novel disease entity that affects an estimated 10% of most populations. ATI sensitivity can explain many symptoms that were thought to be caused by gluten and are still sometimes discussed in public as "gluten-sensitivity". ATI are found in gluten-containing cereals, but they are a completely different class of proteins. Surprisingly, nutritional ATI exacerbate chronic diseases. These diseases are usually diseases outside the intestine. Intestinal discomfort and abdominal pain are no characteristics of ATI-sensitivity, as one might expect. Rather, ATI promote autoimmune diseases, such as multiple sclerosis, rheumatoid arthritis, and lupus, but also worsen metabolic disorders, such as obesity, type 2 diabetes and non-alcoholic steatohepatitis (NASH)—diseases of modern life. We see the striking effects of the ATI-reduced diet in the majority of our patients with these diseases. We give detailed instructions for the ATI-reduced diet in Chap. 5.

Chapter 7 deals with food allergies, with a special focus on the newly discovered *atypical food allergies*. While symptoms of *classical food allergies* are well known, they are relatively rare. They usually manifest with an immediate reaction, such as itching, sneezing, watery eyes, or severe life-threatening symptoms, like anaphylactic shock. In contrast, *atypical* wheat and other food allergies are far more frequent, affecting up to 10% of most populations, and cause mainly abdominal symptoms,

© Springer Nature Switzerland AG 2019
D. Schuppan, K. Gisbert-Schuppan, *Wheat Syndromes*
https://doi.org/10.1007/978-3-030-19023-1_1

such as bloating, pain, diarrhea, or constipation. These symptoms are remarkably similar to the symptoms of irritable bowel syndrome (IBS). In fact, most patients with IBS have an identifiable atypical food allergy, prominently to wheat, and become symptom-free once the allergen is excluded. We have developed an endoscopic technique to directly demonstrate this food allergy in the small intestine, but also describe a more practicable path to identify the allergen. In contrast to classical allergies, in atypical food allergies, it may take many hours until the symptoms become apparent. It is this insidious nature of the atypical food allergies that makes allergen identification difficult without appropriate guidance.

Apart from the novel entities, ATI-sensitivity and atypical food allergies, we devote an in-depth chapter on celiac disease (Chap. 4). Celiac disease is an outstanding example of a disease in which a defined nutrient, gluten from wheat and related cereals, causes intestinal inflammation in patients with a genetic predisposition. The term "celiac disease" is well known to a broad public, but only a few understand the underlying mechanisms and their clinical manifestations. Instead of expected abdominal symptoms like diarrhea and belly pain, most patients with celiac disease have atypical symptoms that manifest in other organs than the gut. Therefore, the majority of celiacs, up to 90%, remains undetected, even in countries with a well-developed healthcare system. The overall prevalence of celiac disease is about 1% in most populations. Once diagnosed, its treatment is straightforward: The rigorous exclusion of even traces of gluten-containing foods. Still, some patients may not improve on the gluten-free diet, since they have developed a severe form, called "refractory celiac disease", or even celiac disease-related intestinal lymphoma. With a highly reliable blood test—anti-tissue transglutaminase antibodies—most celiacs can be identified. Early diagnosis of celiac disease is particularly important for infants and children, in order to secure a normal development and prevent complications.

Due to its overrepresentation in public, we add a chapter on the so-called FODMAPs (fermentable oligo-, di-, monosaccharides, and polyols). These are natural constituents of most foods. When consumed in excess, they can cause bloating, sometimes also abdominal pain and diarrhea in some people. These effects are long known to humankind. Examples are onions, cabbage, beans, watermelon, and other fruits and vegetables. They are non-inflammatory; in contrast, they promote a healthy gut (Chaps. 5, 6, and 10). In Chap. 6 we also touch the common sugar intolerances for lactose and fructose that can cause similar symptoms as FODMAPs and are equally non-inflammatory. These intolerances are usually mild and do not justify the rigorous exclusion of foods containing lactose or fructose. Often these diagnostic labels prevent the search for the inflammatory diseases that we discuss in this book. Finally, we discuss histamine intolerance that rarely presents in a severe form and is often equally overrated.

The book concludes with a chapter in which we present the concept of our unique patient care that we have established in our outpatient clinic (Chap. 9). Thus, we carry out an in-depth exploration, which includes an extensive history taking, a meticulous study of the prior medical records, a thorough physical examination, and consideration of the patient's psycho-social context. Only after this workup, we add missing diagnostic studies and develop a therapeutic plan. This is very time-consuming and currently not adequately reimbursed by health insurance, although it usually markedly helps the patients who are finally cured of their disease that had forced them to have numerous consultations and unnecessary tests and procedures before. Finally, our approach will lead to a dramatic reduction of healthcare costs incurred by mis- and under-diagnosis of the here described highly prevalent food-related inflammatory diseases.

All information that we provide in this book is largely based on our scientific results that have been published in the best scientific and medical journals. Selected original articles and reviews can be found in our annotated bibliography at the end of the book. Our scientific work goes hand in hand with our clinical practice. Therefore, we present individual patients and their disease and treatment process in each of the three major clinical chapters.[1] A subsequent medical commentary on every individual case helps to build an in-depth understanding of the diseases.

---

[1] All histories and aspects reflect true cases from our clinical practice. Nonetheless, the cases we present are completely anonymized, i.e., cases have been modified not to allow identification of the individual person.

Chapter 2
Wheat, Gluten and ATI: An Overview

2.1 A Brief History of Wheat

Wheat is the world's no. 1 staple food and has left rice and corn far behind. Meanwhile, countries that are not spontaneously associated with wheat, such as China and India, have the highest production and consumption worldwide alongside the EU. Therefore, we present some in-depth information about wheat and related cereals that have become our most popular staple food (Fig. 2.1).

Historically, wheat was systematically cultivated in Mesopotamia, today's Middle East, for the first time. Previously, it was ancestral wheat that grew wild and was certainly also used by gatherers and hunters as food, but naturally in small quantities. From Mesopotamia, wheat cultivation spread to England and Western Europe, but also Africa and Egypt, over the next millennia. Wheat was probably first cultivated in most of Europe about 6000 years ago (Fig. 2.2).

The original form of wheat is einkorn (triticum), a wild wheat with a diploid set of chromosomes, i.e., there are two equal sets of chromosomes as in all somatic cells of higher organisms. By crossing-in goat grass into einkorn emmer-wheat was created, a tetraploid wheat with four chromosomes. Durum wheat is related to this ancient tetraploid wheat and is still used to produce today's pasta and other Italian wheat products. The hexaploid wheat, whose early form is spelt, was created approximately 3000 years ago by further crossbreeding. The modern bread wheat variants are all further developments of this hexaploid wheat. Today there is a large number of hexaploid wheat varieties, depending on the country and region, that have been created by breeding for storm resilience, high yield and pest resistance (Figs. 2.3 and 2.4).

These breedings have influenced the nutrient and gluten content. Targeted genetic manipulation does not play any role in the described changes in wheat. Barley and rye are also related to wheat and contain storage proteins similar to gluten. Therefore, patients with coeliac disease are not allowed to eat them any more than wheat. Like wheat, barley and rye also contain ATI. Among our popular domestic cereals, corn

© Springer Nature Switzerland AG 2019
D. Schuppan, K. Gisbert-Schuppan, *Wheat Syndromes*
https://doi.org/10.1007/978-3-030-19023-1_2

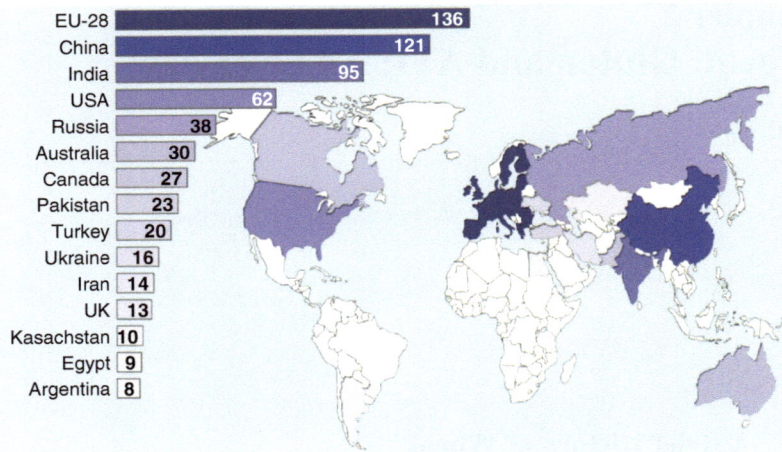

Fig. 2.1 Worldwide wheat cultivation. Wheat has become the most important staple in most countries. Main wheat producers are China and the EU, followed by India, the US and Russia. These main producers are also the top consumers. Numbers are million tons per year

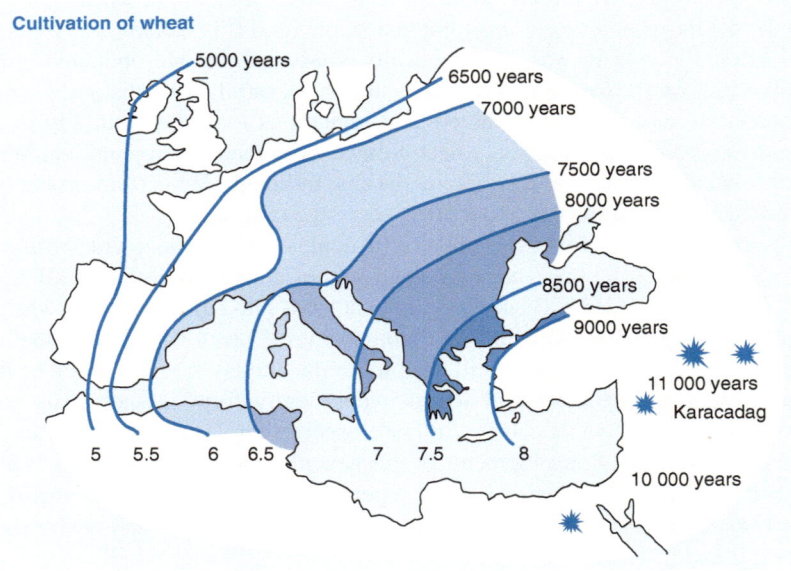

Fig. 2.2 The spread of wheat cultivation. First evidence of systematic wheat cultivation almost 11,000 years ago has been discovered in the village of Karacadag in Eastern Turkey. Shortly afterwards wheat was farmed in Mesopotamia (today's Iraq), Syria and Egypt. Early cultivated wheats were einkorn (diploid set of chromosomes), emmer and durum (both with tetraploid, i.e., a duplicated set of chromosomes). These earlier wheats are still closely related to wild wheat. However, more modern wheats (hexaploid, three sets of chromosomes) were found that were cultivated already 8300 years ago. Bread making was particularly refined in ancient Egypt. It took several thousand years until wheat cultivation reached central Europe and finally the British isles

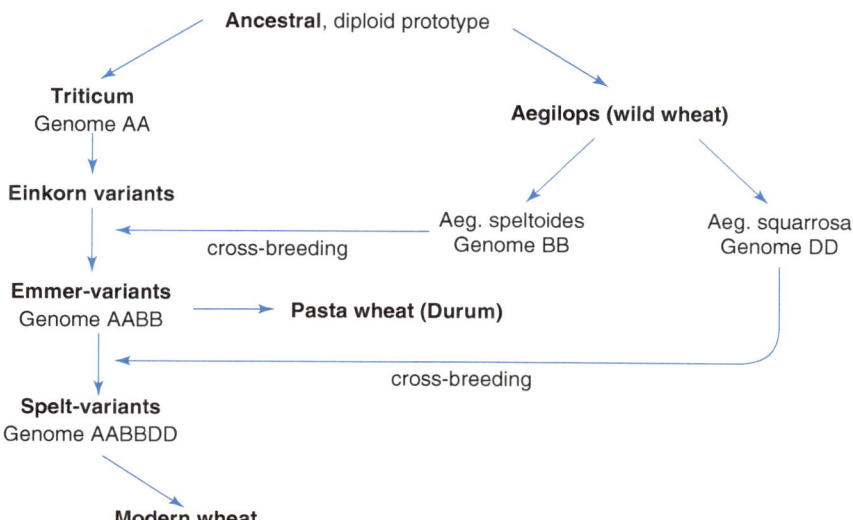

Fig. 2.3 Generation of modern wheat by cross-breeding. Einkorn (triticum), the earliest wheat variant whose cultivation today is very limited due to low yield, low weather and pest resistance, has a diploid set of chromosomes (AA). By crossing in of another diploid wheat, this set was duplicated yielding tetraploid wheat AABB) and finally triplicated (AABBDD). Emmer und hard wheat (pasta or durum wheat) are tetraploid, spelt and modern bread wheat are hexaploid

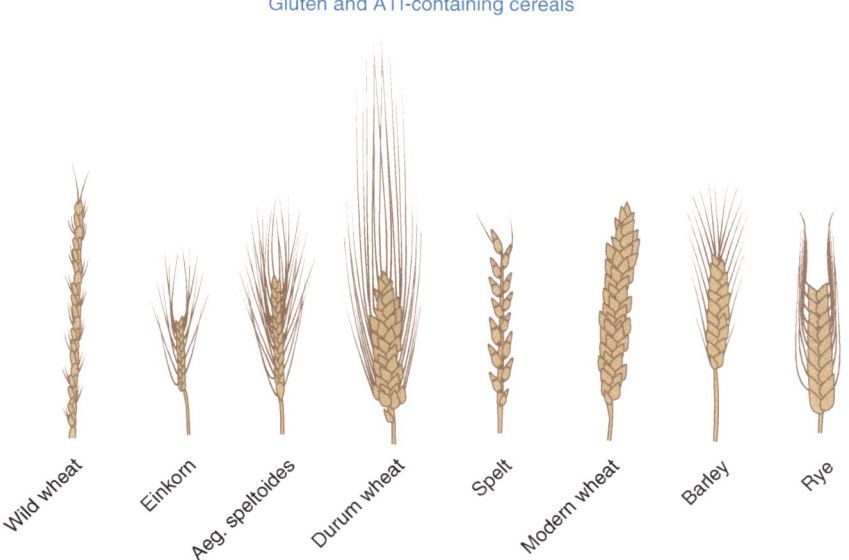

Fig. 2.4 Gluten- and ATI-containing grains. Illustration of the archetypical (wild), the cultivated diploid, tetraploid and modern hexaploid wheats, including the related rye and barley

and oats are not related to wheat. Accordingly, they contain neither ATI nor gluten. However, coeliac patients must be careful when consuming rolled oats because these are often cross-contaminated with gluten-containing cereals during the milling processes.

2.2 What is Gluten?

The nutrients in the wheat grain primarily provide the energy needed for germination and the building blocks to allow the wheat plant to grow. The main energy source is starch that is stored and converted into glucose as needed (Fig. 2.5).

Gluten in particular, but also other proteins, are used to support the growth of the seedling. Only the proteins play a role in wheat-related diseases. Proteins account for 8–13% of the dry weight of the wheat grain and flour. Gluten is predominant

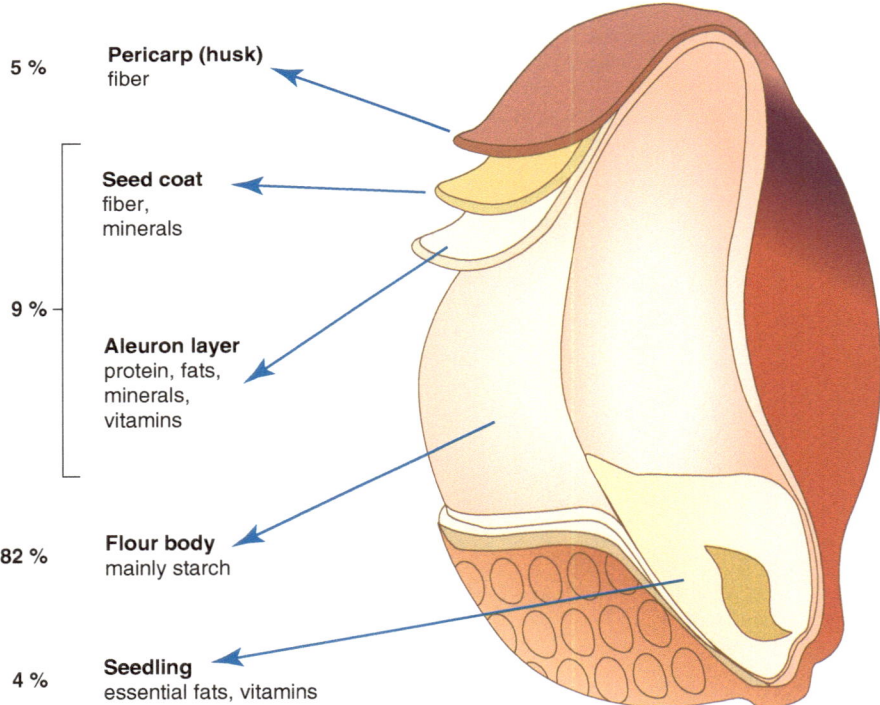

Fig. 2.5 Structure of the wheat grain. The proteins of wheat (rye, barley) can cause celiac disease, wheat allergy and ATI- sensitivity. They are found in the aleurone layer of the grain, ATI also in the endosperm. The endosperm provides energy stored as starch, while gluten serves as protein source for the growing seedling, and ATI regulate the availability of both starch and gluten as energy and protein source, respectively

with 80–90% of total wheat protein. Gluten forms a large family of chain-like molecules with a chain-length of roughly 200–600 amino acids.

The proteins in the human body are made up of about 20 different amino acids. In gluten, two amino acids predominate, namely proline and glutamine. Proline and glutamine cause an unusual protein structure. Due to this unusual structure, human enzymes cannot fully degrade—meaning: digest—gluten proteins. Therefore, about 10% of the gluten consumed remains in the form of protein fragments, the so-called gluten peptides. These gluten peptides are partially absorbed by the intestinal mucosa. In celiac patients, they activate the immune cells of the intestine. This activation does not occur in healthy subjects, as detailed below. Healthy people simply excrete these undigested peptides, e.g., in the urine. If the gluten peptides were completely broken down into their amino acid components, the gluten would not exert its pathogenic effect in celiacs. The complete digestion of gluten peptides is currently evaluated as a novel therapy for celiac disease. Gluten endows the dough with highly valued properties, such as a light and firm texture at the same time, thus being considered essential for the palatability of baked food products. Without gluten, the dough would not rise and would not become light and soft on the inside and crispy on the outside.

The gluten proteins that are so important for the baking properties are divided into two sub-groups, namely gliadins and glutenins (Fig. 2.6). During the baking

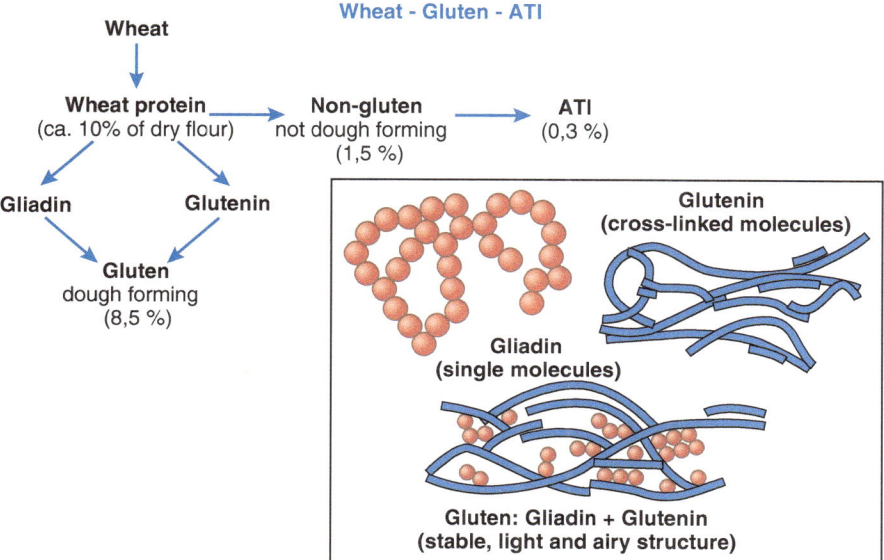

Fig. 2.6 Gluten and non-gluten proteins. Gluten is the main wheat protein, representing about 10% of the flour dry weight. It is a mixture of several gliadin and glutenin proteins that together form high molecular weight structures that endow bread and other bakery products with the desired airy texture, a crispy crust and palatability. 85–90% of the wheat protein is gluten. The other 10–15% non-gluten proteins consist of numerous different molecules that play important roles in the regulation of the energy, lipid and protein metabolism of the grain, determine its development, growth and germination towards the wheat plant. ATI represent only 3% of wheat protein and 0.3% of flour dry weight

process, glutenins form higher sponge-like structures by cross-linking that lead to the desired airy softness in the final baking product. The gliadins contribute by stabilizing the cavities and the net-like structure. These sponge-like structures store water and carbon dioxide, particularly well during cooking and baking. For a long time, it was assumed that only the gliadins cause coeliac disease and that their elimination by genetic engineering of the wheat genome would enable coeliac patients to consume wheat products without developing symptoms. However, these attempts were futile, since firstly, gliadins significantly contribute to the good baking properties of gluten and secondly, glutenins also cause celiac disease. For this reason, a separate discussion of glutenins and gliadins, as can still be found in scientific and medical articles, is not needed.

2.3   What are ATI?

Besides gluten, wheat also contains hundreds of other proteins. However, these only make up 10–15% of the total wheat protein. Among these proteins are several enzymes that play a role in grain germination, for example, amylases and proteases. Moreover, there are proteins that inhibit these enzymes. These non-gluten proteins include amylase trypsin inhibitors—ATI. There is little research about the function of the ATI. We are sure that they regulate the process of wheat germination and that they protect the storage carbohydrates (starch) and the storage protein (gluten) from premature degradation by inhibiting the amylase enzymes and the trypsin-like proteases. Amylases break down the starch into glucose that provides the most important source of energy available for the seedling. The trypsin-like proteases split the gluten proteins into single amino acids or small peptides that the grain needs to germinate and to produce the early stages of the plant.

   While amylases and trypsin are also enzymes of the human digestive tract, their specificity and activity are different from the wheat enzymes. Therefore, ATI do not inhibit the human enzymes as potently as the wheat enzymes. Unexpectedly, ATI have another serious effect in the mammalian and therefore human intestinal tract, since they induce inflammation. This is the cause of ATI-sensitivity as we describe in detail in Chap. 5.

Chapter 3
Immunology of the Intestine

3.1 Our Largest Immune Organ: The Intestine

The intestine harbors our largest immune organ and therefore plays a decisive role in maintaining a healthy state of the entire body. It is a gatekeeper and a central mediator of the body's interaction with the life-sustaining, but also potentially harmful environment. A basic understanding of the essential immunological processes in the intestine is very helpful for a deeper insight into cereal-related diseases. Therefore, we present the multi-layered structure of the intestine and the function of the embedded cells in detail. An overview of the digestive organs is given in Fig. 3.1.

3.2 Anatomy of an All-Rounder

To maximize its surface, the intestine has microscopic finger-like protrusions, the so-called intestinal villi, alternating with microscopic dips and "valleys", the so called intestinal crypts. The villi are particularly pronounced in the small intestine, which is responsible for the absorption of nutrients. With a surface area of between 200 and 300 m² (22,000 to 33,000 ft²) in adults, the intestine is also the largest immune organ. The surface of the human skin, the second largest immune organ, is between 1.5 and 2.3 m² (16.5 to 17.5 ft²) in adults. The respiratory tract with nasopharynx, trachea, and lungs only takes third position among the immune organs that interact with the outside world. These three organ systems, unlike the other major organs, are in constant contact and exchange with the outside world. They are lined with mucous membranes that must be permeable to substances from the outside world, in order to absorb vital substances. On the other hand, they must ensure that harmful influences are fended off immediately before they can enter and possibly damage the internal organs. This is a highly complex task, as we are all constantly

© Springer Nature Switzerland AG 2019
D. Schuppan, K. Gisbert-Schuppan, *Wheat Syndromes*
https://doi.org/10.1007/978-3-030-19023-1_3

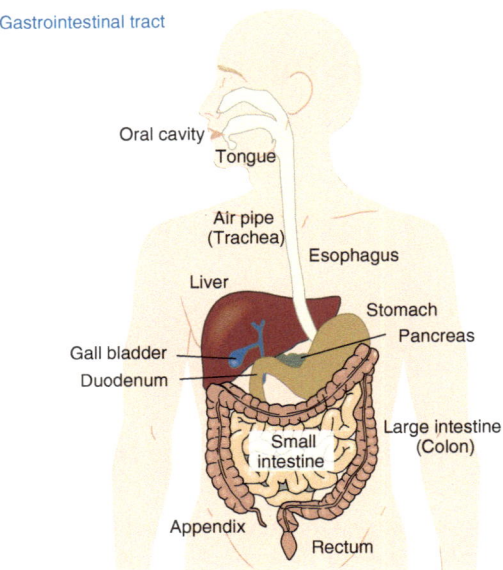

Fig. 3.1 The digestive system. The food is crushed, wetted and mixed in the oral cavity. Predigestion of starch is started with the enzyme amylase in the oral cavity. Swallowing transports the slurry via the esophagus into the stomach that serves as reservoir to further mix and digest the mash with the protein cleaving enzyme pepsin. The acidic milieu of the stomach also curtails the multiplication of harmful bacteria. In the upper part of the small intestine, immediately after the stomach (duodenum), pancreatic juice neutralizes the stomach acid. The pancreas also produces and secretes the central enzymes needed for a thorough digestion, of carbohydrates, lipids, proteins and nucleic acids, which allows their resorption in the 4–5 m (13–16 ft) long small intestine. The epithelial cells that cover the small intestine are equipped with cell-bound enzymes that cleave especially dimeric sugars (disaccharides such as household sugar) into resorbable monosaccharides and small peptides into resorbable single amino acids. Monosaccharides, amino acids and single nucleic acids produced by nucleases are then actively taken up by the intestinal epithelial cells and handed over into small blood vessels (capillaries) of the lamina propria (see below). From the capillaries that collect into larger blood vessels they reach the liver mainly via the portal vein as well as other organs and regions of the body. Nutritional fats are cleaved into smaller molecules by lipases after their emulsification by bile acids that are produced in the liver and stored in the gall bladder that extrudes the bile acids via the bile duct into the duodenum once the food has entered the small intestine. In the intestinal epithelial cells the lipid constituents like fatty acids, glycerol and cholesterol are assembled to large lipid vesicles (the chylomicrons) that are also carried to the liver via the bloodstream. The liver reassembles these lipids and exports them as, e.g., high or low density lipoprotein particles that circulate in the blood to supply other tissues. Most minerals and vitamins are resorbed in the proximal (upper), some such as vitamin B12, in the distal (lower) small intestine. The nutrient passage from proximal to distal takes about 2 h, while the density of the symbiotic microbes in the intestinal contents increases from 1000 to 100 million/ml (10^8). In the ileum and more so in the colon bacterial density further increases up to 1000 billion (10^{12}). In the colon, otherwise nondigestable plant-derived carbohydrates are fermented by the abundant microbial flora, producing gases like carbon dioxide and methane, but also short chain fatty acids that nourish and protect the gut epithelial cells. In the colon, also minerals are exchanged and the water is removed from the remnant food mash that becomes more and more replaced by the symbiotic gut bacteria and finally excreted as feces. It is plausible that, given these complexities, disturbances or a disbalance in every section of the digestive system, be it motility, the function of digestive enzymes, nutrient uptake, reassembly and transport, or colonization with a pathological microbiota (dysbiosis) can lead to severe disturbances, malaise and disease inside and outside of the intestine

exposed to the most diverse influences from our environment. Just think of the many bacteria and viruses with which we come into contact in everyday life, but which are usually successfully fended off by all three organ systems and prevented from getting entry into the body's interior.

How is this complex task even possible, especially for the intestine? Lungs and skin are basically only focused on the exchange of oxygen for carbon-dioxide. In contrast, the intestine permits us to consume and resorb a tremendous variety of foods and therefore potentially harmful constituents and molecules without being even disturbed, let alone in a constant inflammatory state. This discriminatory ability of the intestine is unique and results from a pre-structured highly specialized and complex immune system that, in addition, needs the above mentioned early learning processes. It is a virtual miracle that many of us have a healthy gut that has developed these immune regulatory processes.

3.3 An Organ in the Organ: The Intestinal Microbiome

The intestine itself is not only a functionally and anatomically independent organ but is also the home of another organ, one that has only recently been recognized and whose far-reaching significance for the human body and brain is just being deciphered: the intestinal microbiome. The intestinal microbiome mainly comprises the useful intestinal bacteria that support the intestinal tract to digest food. However, it may also comprise bacteria that may have negative effects on the body, but these bacteria are normally kept in check by their useful counterparts that are called commensal bacteria. The intestinal bacteria mass is approximately 1.5 kg (3,3 lb). This makes it our largest internal organ that is even larger than the liver. In total, it contains up to 1000 trillion (one quadrillion = 10^{15}) bacteria, up to 30 times as many as we carry body cells in us. The density of intestinal microbes is low at about 1000 bacteria/mL in the upper small intestine, but increases rapidly in the course of the 4–5 m long small intestine to reach about 1 billion/mL (10^9) in the ileum that is the end part of the small intestine. The highest bacterial concentration is found at the end of the approximately 1 m long large intestine with 1 trillion/mL (10^{12}). Since most of these microorganisms are useful bacteria, the intestine has learned to recognize them as friends. It has gone through a similar learning process to recognize food as harmless. On the other hand, it can quickly recognize and start to fend off unfamiliar food components and especially bacteria or viruses as foreign invaders. This highly complex task of distinguishing between friend and foe is carried out by the intestinal immune system.

3.4 Immune Cells in the Intestine

The intestinal wall is composed of seven characteristic layers (Fig. 3.2). From the inside out, these are

1. the epithelial layer facing the intestinal contents,
2. the first layer of connective tissue underneath,

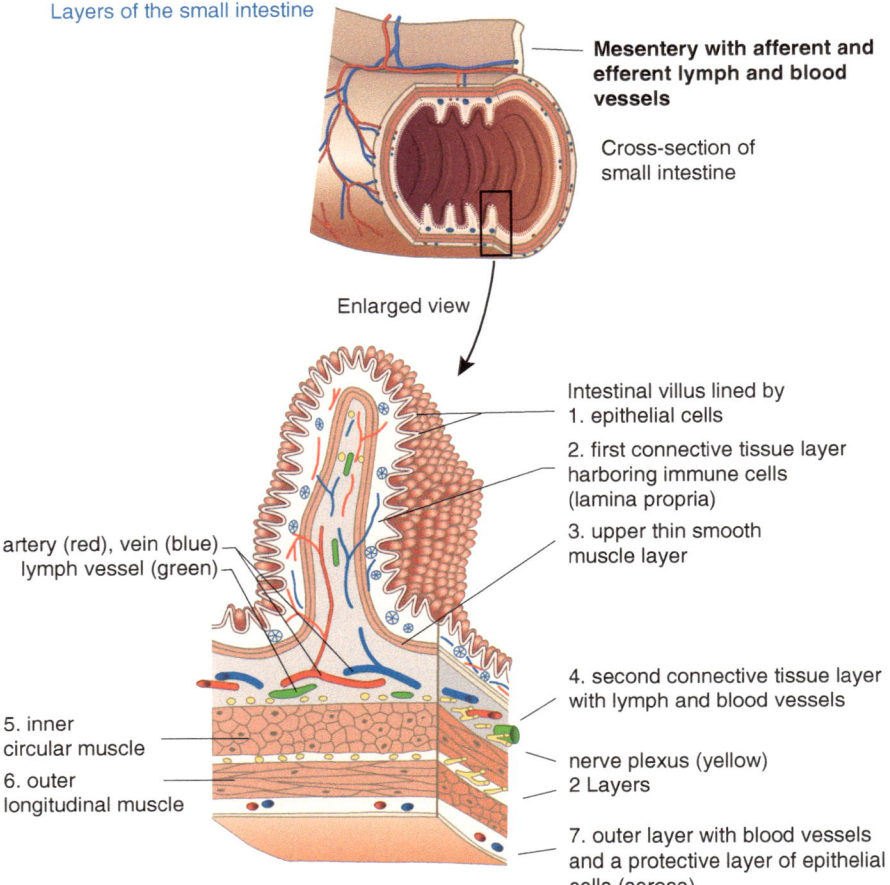

Layers of the small intestine

Mesentery with afferent and efferent lymph and blood vessels

Cross-section of small intestine

Enlarged view

Intestinal villus lined by 1. epithelial cells

2. first connective tissue layer harboring immune cells (lamina propria)

3. upper thin smooth muscle layer

artery (red), vein (blue) lymph vessel (green)

4. second connective tissue layer with lymph and blood vessels

5. inner circular muscle

nerve plexus (yellow) 2 Layers

6. outer longitudinal muscle

7. outer layer with blood vessels and a protective layer of epithelial cells (serosa)

Fig. 3.2 Layers of the intestine. The intestine is attached to other organs via the mesentery, a connective tissue that also harbors the blood vessels that supply the gut with oxygen and nutrients (arteries) or carry the resorbed nutrients towards the liver and other organs. The lymph vessels transport the resorbed fats as small lipid vesicles (chylomicrons). The inner surface of the intestine is dramatically enlarged by protrusions of the mucosa called villi. This secures an efficient uptake of nutrients. The intestinal epithelial cells constitute the inner intestinal lining of the gut. They are firmly anchored to the first layer of connective tissue (lamina propria). This thin layer harbors the major portion of the intestinal immune system and smaller blood vessels (capillaries), and is attached to a thin layer of smooth muscle on the other side that can move the villi, to further increase the contact with nutrients. This is followed by another layer of connective tissue that contains larger blood vessels and lymphatics that are connected to the liver and other organs via the blood vessels of the mesentery. The circular and longitudinal smooth muscle layers of the gut are activated by an inner and an outer nerve plexus within the autonomous nervous system. The extensions of these nerves sense pain and expansion of the gut wall, and react by inducing either contraction or relaxation of smooth muscle. The outer sheath of the gut is made up of the serosa, a protective layer of connective tissue and epithelium that also contains blood vessels that communicate with the mesentery and the rest of the body

3. an underlying thin muscle layer which moves the intestinal villi,
4. a second connective tissue layer which carries blood and lymph vessels,
5. a transverse muscle layer,
6. a longitudinal muscle layer, and
7. finally, the layer of epithelial cells that enwraps the intestine and that faces the abdominal cavity (Fig. 3.2).

The intestinal immune system is located in the middle of the intestinal wall and consists of a large number of different immune cells. Overall, the intestinal wall is very thin. It has a thickness of 2–3 mm in the healthy small intestine and 3–5 mm in the healthy large intestine. The first layer, the epithelium that faces the intestinal contents consists only of a single layer of cells. The epithelial cells are about 20 µm high. They sit very close to each other and usually only allow very small molecules to pass through, namely, the degraded food components, water, and electrolytes. However, even these are not simply waved through, but are selectively transported by special mechanisms. Specialized intestinal epithelial cells, the M cells, also actively take up small amounts of larger molecules that are then presented to tolerance-inducing immune cells beneath. This is an important way for the intestine to learn to which molecules it should react with tolerance. In the case of inflammation in the intestine, e.g., during viral or bacterial infections, larger molecules can increasingly flow into the immune cell layer. In this case, tolerance against food-derived molecules that were previously sensed as harmless can be broken. We come back to this important mechanism in of our clinical cases, one with celiac disease and one with chronic inflammatory bowel disease. The epithelial cells have another important function. They produce a protective layer, the mucus or mucin layer, covering the inside of the intestine that among other things hampers the penetration of bacteria from the intestinal contents into the intestinal wall and thus the whole body.

The layer on which the epithelium rests is a layer of connective tissue. It contains tiny blood vessels that connect the intestinal vascular system to that of all other organs. These tiny blood vessels transport the small molecular nutrients that have been absorbed by the epithelial cells to the other organs and primarily to the liver. Most importantly, this layer harbors most of the immune cells of the intestine and thus a large part of the immune cells of the entire body.

Below this "immune layer" lies a thin muscle layer that moves the intestinal villi to improve nutrient transport and uptake. Below is a wider layer of connective tissue that carries the larger blood and lymph vessels. These vessels ultimately transport the nutrients into the liver. This is followed by the longitudinal and the circular muscle layer. A thin layer of connective tissue and a one-layered epithelium, the so-called serosa, finally ensheathes the whole intestine. The circular muscle induces intestinal contractions, i.e., mixes the food components, whereas the longitudinal musculature transports the food and later also the feces from top to bottom. All contractions in the intestine are essentially autonomously controlled by the nervous system of the gastrointestinal tract. They are therefore largely independent of conscious processes. This makes the gastrointestinal tract the largest nervous organ after the brain. Interestingly, all neurotransmitters, i.e., those substances that regulate nerve transmission in the brain, are also found in the intestine. On the other hand, nerve hormones that were first discovered in the intestine later were also found in the brain. In this respect, the intestine can also be seen as an external branch of the brain—or the brain likewise as an external branch of the intestine.

Taken together, the intestinal wall is constructed in such a way that the immune cells in the upper connective tissue layer are in contact with both the blood vessels and the nervous system. Thus, all immune cell processes that are linked to the intestinal contents (food and microbiota) always also influence the activity of the intestinal nerves and muscles. In addition, they affect all organs outside the intestine through the blood system via the release of mediators (messenger molecules) and through nerve signaling. Overall, all processes and events in the intestine have effects on the entire organism (see Fig. 3.3). The multifaceted anatomical, immuno-

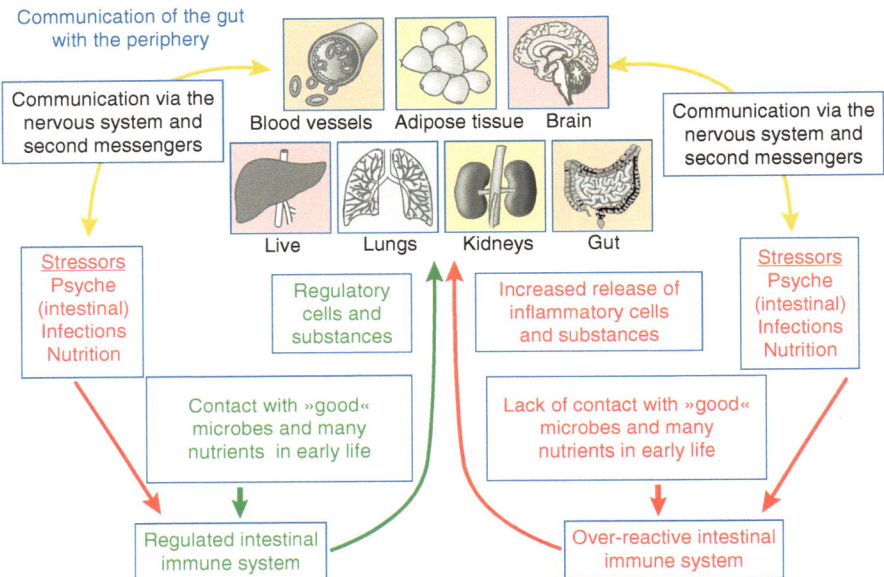

Fig. 3.3 Communication of the intestine with the periphery. The gut is the organ with the largest surface exposed to the environment. Even more than the skin, the immune system of the gut must discriminate between the enormous quantity of useful nutrients that it also has to resorb actively and the beneficial commensal microbiota, and a few potentially dangerous molecules, bacteria and viruses. The intestine's learning process to discriminate between "friend" and "foe" begins with birth when the newborn is exposed to the mother's and other environmental microbes, as well as to oral nutrients, initially the mother's milk, for the first time. The confrontation with other usually harmless environmental stimuli, e.g., pollen or certain bacteria, via the mucous membranes of the airways, or with common antigens and commensal bacteria to which the skin is exposed promotes this learning process to acquire an adequate immune tolerance. Gaps during this educational process, as occur in highly sanitized environments, are with frequent antibiotic treatments, appear to favor allergies and autoimmune diseases. This has been plausibly put forward by the so-called hygiene hypothesis that stresses these adverse consequences of too much hygiene. Inflammatory signals from the gut are not only limited to the digestive organs but also affect inflammation in extraintestinal, peripheral organs, including the brain. In turn, nerve signals and blood-borne factors from the brain affect the function and inflammation in the gut

logical and neurological interactions, as demonstrated here, underline the relevance of holistic approaches in health and disease. Any reductionist approach to disease would necessarily neglect the complexity of the human body and compromise the quality of treatment. The non-trivial consequences of this view for clinical practice are discussed in Chap. 9.

3.5   Complexity of the Immune System

The functioning of the immune system is extraordinarily complex. Numerous novel scientific reports are published every day that add formerly unknown aspects to our understanding. Our presentation in this chapter goes beyond classical textbook knowledge, but results from our longstanding, continuous study of this very complicated system. Results from our own scientific research projects as well as the ongoing exchange with research colleagues and cooperation partners worldwide have contributed. The extraordinary complexity of the immune system results from the networks of feedback loops that interact with each other and can mutually reinforce or counteract each other. One aim of these mechanisms is to maximize the immune system's defensive function in order to protect the organism in the best possible way, without harming the body. The compensatory mechanisms are so effective that a single malfunction can usually be attenuated immediately, thus preventing serious consequences for the organism. The immune system is not easily thrown out of balance. A general dysbalance, such as chronic illness, only occurs when the finely tuned immune system has been challenged by a large number of repetitive hits that cause a worsening maladaptation. In this context, maladaptation means that the immune response becomes inadequate and moves away from equilibrium. Only few years ago, a euphoria prevailed when highly potent drugs were developed that shut down or activated a single signalling pathway as a cure to chronic diseases. However, in most cases these treatments were inefficient or fraught with side effects. This disappointing outcome might have been avoided if the multifaceted fine-tuning of the immune response would have been taken into account. The usually impressive stability of the immune system is based, among other things, upon the two major arms or branches of the immune system.

3.6   Two Arms of the Immune System: Key to Intestinal Health

To defend itself, the body uses two arms of the immune system. They functionally differ significantly, but also complement each other: The innate and the acquired—or adaptive—immune system (Fig. 3.4). The innate immune system plays a decisive role in immediate protection against foreign intruders or harmful substances. It mainly includes the immune cells of the upper intestinal connective tissue layer. These immune cells are equipped with sensors on their surface that detect harmful

Immunology of the Gut

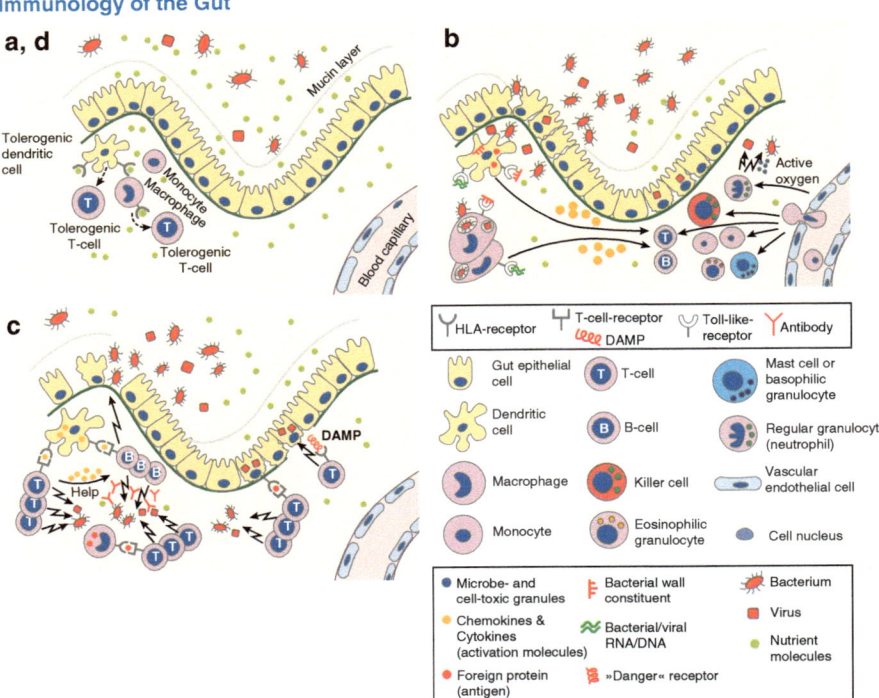

Fig. 3.4 The intestinal immune system. (**a**) State of immune equilibrium—tolerance. Each individual intestinal epithelial cell enlarges its surface towards the gut lumen with miniscule membrane protrusions, the microvilli. The microvilli are covered by a protective mucus layer that is produced by the epithelial cells and that is severalfold higher than the epithelium itself. The epithelial cells are connected with each other on all sides by so-called tight and occlusive junctions. These tight connections together with the mucus layer allow only small molecules (green dots), e.g. nutrient molecules that have been thoroughly digested by pancreatic enzymes, to get access to the surface of the intestinal epithelial cells, but prevent larger molecules, viruses and bacteria to pass. These mechanisms are the basis for an intact intestinal barrier. The epithelial cells further degrade these small nutrient molecules or transform them into other molecules that are utilized by the body. This occurs already at the epithelial surface, when sugars (disaccharides) are further cleaved into monosaccharides by membrane-bound enzymes like lactase or saccharase, when peptides are processed to amino acids by peptidases, or when partly digested lipids are resorbed and later transfromed intracellularly into the body's own lipids and lipid vesicles (chylomicrons) by lipid transferases. The nutrients are carried by specific transporters or within vesicles and exported to the other (abluminal) side of the resorbing epithelial cell to underlying small blood vessels (capillaries) or lymph vessels (for the lipid vesicles) and from there to larger blood vessels in the mesentery (the connective tissue by which the intestine is attached to the other abdominal organs) and finally to the liver and other organs. Even during immune balance, some larger nutrient molecules, mainly peptides from proteins that remained partly undigested, reach the first connective tissue layer that harbors most of the intestinal immune system (the lamina propria). These peptides are large enough to be ingested by antigen presenting cells (mainly dendritic cells, macrophages and monocytes, but also B lymphocytes that recirculate peptides of at least nine amino acids length to their cell surface and present them to T cells via HLA (human leukocyte antigen) molecules. These antigen presenting cells have "learned" not to release mediators (cytokines) that would

attract and activate destructive T cells to proliferate and attack the (food) protein from which the peptide is derived. In contrast, they serve as tolerance-inducing (tolerogenic) cells, whose antigen presentation induces tolerance promoting, so-called regulatory T cells that actively suppress the immune reaction to the foreign protein. This tolerance that has to differentiate between beneficial foreign molecules vs the necessity to raise a quick and effective defense against harmful intruders, is essential for the body's survival. It requires a highly elaborate immune regulation that once tolerance to certain nutrients or usually harmless commensal gut bacteria is brought out of balance can lead to severe inflammation, (**b**) Alarm in the gut—activation of the innate immune system. Harmful bacteria or viruses penetrate and destroy the protective mucin layer. Harmful bacteria may proceed further into the intestinal tissue layers, sometimes also via the capillaries and larger blood vessels into other organs where they can multiply and cause further harm. Under ideal growth conditions bacteria can duplicate every 20 min, a dangerous situation. Viruses often infect and multiply in the intestinal epithelial cells. This can lead to the epithelial cells' death, their shedding from the intestinal lining and further loss of barrier function, which can dramatically increase intestinal permeability. Macrophages and dendritic cells recognize this dangerous invasion via sensors on their surface, the so-called (bacterial, viral) pattern recognition receptors: they ingest (phagocytose) the viruses or bacteria, or larger fragments of them, that are much larger than the usual nutritional molecules that reach the lamina propria. The pattern recognition receptors sense conserved bacterial or viral carbohydrates, lipids, DNA or RNA sequences, or peptides that are different from their mammalian or plant counterparts. Their activation by these danger signals enhances the phagocytotic activity and cytokine release by macrophages and dendritic cells, and also activates other innate immune cells like monocytes and natural killer cells. Within a few minutes after receptor activation, cytokines are released (yellow dots) that diffuse into the surrounding tissue, capillaries and blood vessels to attract more circulating immune cells into the affected intestinal tissue. These are mainly granulocytes, killer lymphocytes, monocytes, T and B lymphocytes. In the intestine the blood-derived monocytes mature to macrophages and dendritic cells further promoting the innate but also paving the way to an adaptive immune response. In case of allergies or a reaction to parasites, the immune response also involves mast cells, eosinophilic and basophilic granulocytes. Activated granulocytes and macrophages also release toxic substances such as reactive oxygen species (oxidizing molecules including oxygen in various active forms, blue dots) that directly kill invaders but also damage the body's own tissue and cells which can cause pain, fever and functional impairment, all signs of acute inflammation. In the gut this manifests as abdominal pain, diarrhea, but also constipation. The scenario resembles a battlefield, with a massive deployment of soldiers armed to the teeth, and an uncertain outcome. (**c**) The second step: activation of adaptive immunity. Now the adaptive immune system comes into play. Its major effectors are the T and B lymphocytes that are attracted to the site of battle by the factors secreted from the activated innate immune cells. Only one out of several thousand T or B lymphocytes bears a receptor on its surface that (by chance during genetic diversification) recognizes a certain bacterial or viral peptide or nonpeptide molecule, or an otherwise harmless, e.g., nutritional molecule (the antigen). This recognition requires presentation of the antigen on the surface of an antigen presenting cell, mainly the dendritic cell and macrophage, via the HLA receptor. Only via this presentation the responding T cell can sense the antigen according to the "key and lock principle" and react by starting to multiply in a process termed clonal expansion. Within a few days the clone army thus generated will consist of millions of identical soldiers, and there will be T cell clones not only directed to a single, but to numerous different antigens, usually from the same single invader, but sometimes also from otherwise harmless "bystanders". During the days of high vulnerability, before the adaptive immune can take over the defense, the innate immune system must keep the infection in check, to prevent the bacteria or viruses from flooding the body, often leading to death. Once the T lymphocytes take over, they start to destroy the invaders in a more effective and specific way, releasing, e.g., toxic molecules, more specifically than the innate immune cells. Apart from the T lymphocytes, antigen specific clones of the B lymphocytes start to multiply. They do not attack the invaders directly, but produce soluble antibodies that similar to the T cell receptors bind to their cognate antigen on the bacterium or virus which blocks their function and activates the complement proteins in the blood that cover the intruder to facilitate its destruction and dissolution by T cells and its phagocytosis by macrophages. For their multiplication and efficient antibody production, the B lymphocytes need help from the T cells that secrete B cell stimulating cytokines. There is a distinctive feature in virus infections. Here the infected (intestinal epithelial) cell can serve as antigen presenting cell, since, different from bacterial infections, the gut pathogenic viruses mainly infect the epithelium. The intestinal epithelial cells can also fulfill other duties of cells of the innate immune system by expressing danger-sensing molecules, "danger associated molecular patterns" (DAMPs), on their surface. These DAMPs are recognized by natural killer lymphocytes that attack and eliminate the virus infected intestinal epithelial cells, as the only way to get rid of the virus. It is easily understandable that this process can lead to severe disease symptoms, such as in viral enteritis. (**d**) The immune system prevails, the cure (*Figure as in a, but with more (memory) lymphocytes*). Fortunately, the sophisticated and highly efficient immune system usually gains control over the infection and to finally eliminate the intruders. In simple virus infection this cure occurs within a few days, maximally 2 weeks. Meanwhile the intestinal epithelium has regenerated, the intercellular junctions have been closed, and the protective mucin layer has been reconstituted. The massively expanded clonal T and to a lesser degree B lymphocyte populations have done their job and, due to the lack of further stimulation by viral (bacterial) antigens by antigen presenting cells, largely undergo apoptosis (cell death). However, a smaller army of these clones remains alive and in reserve, should another attempt of infection by the same microbes occur. In this case, a rapid adaptive (T and B lymphocyte) response can be mounted that can efficiently destroy the invaders before the battle even begins. This memory response is also the basis of prophylactic vaccination using noninfectious viral or bacterial antigens

molecules and react immediately with the release of inflammatory substances that further activate neighboring immune and non-immune cells for defense. They trigger an instant reaction that often leads to elimination of the harmful invaders aiming at preventing them from penetrating into and multiplying in the body. The repertoire of these sensors is relatively limited. Thus, they mainly recognize foreign genetic material or certain cell wall components of bacteria. The cells of the innate immune system that have such sensors are predominantly monocytes, macrophages, dendritic, and natural killer cells. Most other intestinal cells are also equipped with such sensors but to a lower extent.

Even with a strong innate immune reaction, complete elimination of certain pathogens or prevention of their spread in the body is often not possible. Completion of the task often requires the adaptive (acquired) immune system. It is more flexible and destroys the enemy in a much more targeted manner. However, this takes time, as the adaptive cells must first multiply sufficiently, which takes at least a few days. Adaptive cells are mostly lymphocytes that are subdivided into T lymphocytes and B lymphocytes. Activated T lymphocytes destroy the enemies directly, whereas activated B lymphocytes produce antibodies that bind to the intruders and thus inactivate them or promote their destruction by permitting phagocytosis (gobbling up) by macrophages. A large number of lymphocytes circulate in the body with millions of different variants. However, only a small number of each variant is produced. Each of these variants is equipped with different specificity for intruders as defined by their lymphocyte receptor. This secures a high probability that at least one of these lymphocytes will have the right fit to recognize a given intruder.

The different T cell variants are formed at random during cell development. If a specific T cell receptor detects its matching intruder, a signal is propagated to the T lymphocyte nucleus telling the cell to multiply and produce numerous clones of itself that display the same target specificity. The pre-activated lymphocytes are further stimulated when they pass through the lymph nodes where they encounter a large number of so-called antigen presenting cells that carry the target recognition structure of the intruder.

Once massive clonal expansion of the T cells has been achieved, the body has gained adaptive immune control in most cases. This means not only that the acute infection is usually fought off but also that upon renewed infection, even after many years, the primed T lymphocytes can mount a quicker and more effective immediate defense.

Even if a number of T cell clones decreases over the years when no re-stimulation occurs, memory cells remain, which can refresh the old clone army in a very short time. This mechanism of clonal expansion and memory response is exploited for protective vaccination. Here protein fragments of bacteria or viruses are injected into the skin or applied via mucosal membranes (e.g., oral polio vaccination). As detailed below, these proteins are absorbed by the dendritic cells and the macrophages in the skin or the lymph nodes, which present them to the T cells and induce their clonal reproduction. The resulting protection often lasts for years, even when no pathogenic contact takes place, and the number of T cell clones has decreased again.

3.6.1   How Does the T Cell Know When to Expand?

The major cells of the innate immune system, i.e., monocytes, macrophages, and dendritic cells, also take over the function of so-called antigen presenting cells. They phagocytose the intruder or take up parts of it and recirculate fragments of foreign proteins to their surface via specific receptors (so-called human lymphocyte antigens—HLA). The HLA-presented fragments can now be recognized by the specific T cell clone—following the key-lock-principle—to induce their clonal expansion.

This processing of foreign material by the antigen presenting cells is a core part of the adaptive immune response. From an immunological point of view, this process transforms the intruder into "antibody generators", so-called antigens. An antigen is a molecule that triggers a T cell response and induces the production of such an army of T cell clones as well as antibody producing B cell clones. The term antigen, which unfortunately makes one think of genetics, is in fact only an abbreviation for the term "antibody generator". The antibody generating molecules are mainly proteins, but also some carbohydrate structures, lipid molecules, and chemicals. Since many molecules also circulate in the body without being derived from foreign intruders or other harmful sources, the presentation by antigen presenting cells, the first line of defense, is needed to enable the T cell to identify the substance as dangerous. Therefore, presentation on this "silver platter" (HLA-molecule) is required to mount the T cell-mediated immune response.

In this way, with the process of antigen presentation, the innate immune system centrally supports the acquired immune system. In addition to monocytes, macrophages, and dendritic cells, the intestinal epithelial cells also perform an antigen presenting task, namely when they are infected by viruses. In the other three, so-called professional antigen presenting cell types, antigen presentation occurs highly efficiently after phagocytosis or fragment uptake, usually with the destruction of the intruder. Here the dendritic cells are the most effective antigen presenting cells.

Understanding this interaction between the two arms of the immune system is very helpful to comprehend the cereal intolerances described in the following chapters.

3.6.2   How Does the Immune System Develop Tolerance to Food?

How is it possible that this extremely complex defense system, which has to fend off intruders from the outside, is tolerant to the myriads of molecules in the food that we eat and recognizes them as "friends", instead of mounting a strong defensive immune response against them. Scientifically, this is only partly understood. What we know is that there are also antigen presenting cells in the intestine that induce an anti-inflammatory, so-called tolerogenic immune response in T lymphocytes with the help of tolerogenic dendritic cells. They present food antigens in the same way as their inflammation inducing counterparts. But they also secrete factors (cytokines and chemokines) that stimulate the T cells in an opposite way. These T cells also expand, but rather suppress other inflammatory cells; they are called regulatory or suppressor T cells. This means that expansion of these regulatory T cells is both, non-inflammatory and actively suppressing an ongoing inflammatory T cell reaction.

The tolerogenic cells are predominantly found in the so-called lymph follicles that are located at specialized sites underneath the M cells. The M cells are a particular subset of intestinal epithelial cells with an increased permeability for small peptides and molecules.

3.6.3   What is the "Leaky Gut"?

Permeability of the intestinal epithelium for larger protein fragments is necessary to maintain tolerance to harmless molecules from the environment. These fragments reach the lamina propria (the first layer of connective tissue, see Fig. 3.2) and thus the intestinal immune system. In the case of intestinal inflammation, an excess of inflammatory mediators (proteins and small molecules that further activate the immune cells, mainly cytokines and chemokines) is released. These mediators increase intestinal permeability, i.e., leakiness. This occurs via an opening of inter-epithelial cell contacts creating gaps that permit the entry of even larger molecules into the lamina propria on the one hand (para-cellular transport). On the other hand, it leads to an increase of active transport of molecules from the luminal to the basal side of the epithelium (trans-cellular transport). Both mechanisms lead to more influx of molecules into the major immune compartment of the gut. It is obvious that permeability can be massively increased in severe intestinal inflammations, as is found in active celiac disease, in inflammatory bowel disease (Crohn's disease, ulcerative colitis) or in acute bacterial or viral enteritis. A slight increase in perme-ability is also found in irritable bowel syndrome that also has an inflammatory com-ponent. When the acute inflammatory stimulus subsides, the increased para-cellular and trans-cellular transport quickly (within one to a few hours) returns to baseline. Except for very rare genetic diseases, there is no evidence of a so-called "leaky gut" as an inborn predisposition for chronic disease. In contrast, the "leaky gut" is rather a consequence of intestinal inflammation due to other causes.

Chapter 4
Celiac Disease and its Manifold Manifestations

4.1 What is Celiac Disease?

For a long time, only those affected knew what gluten and celiac disease were all about. In recent years, however, gluten-free food is sold in virtually every supermarket. Hollywood stars and other celebrities are publicly promoting the gluten-free diet, and the mass media are increasingly taking up the subject in talk shows, documentaries, and commentaries. Almost everyone has come into contact with the idea of a gluten-free diet. It is precisely the public attention that leads to gluten-free food being defended by some with fervor and being disqualified by others as a fad or zeitgeist phenomenon. Marginalized or even ignored in this dispute are those who are affected most, namely patients with celiac disease. In fact, they are the ones who depend on a strictly, that is 100% gluten-free diet and have no other choice. What is celiac disease, and how does it relate to gluten?

4.1.1 Inflammation of the Intestine

Celiac disease is a serious inflammatory bowel disease. The small intestine of those affected reacts with a permanent and pronounced inflammation to dietary gluten. This often leads to the intestine losing its ability to resorb nutrients, resulting in serious nutrient deficiencies and symptoms like chronic anemia, osteoporosis, or damage to the nervous system. The genetic predisposition for celiac disease (HLA-DQ2/DQ8) also predisposes for various autoimmune diseases. These include type 1 diabetes, rheumatic arthritis, autoimmune thyroid diseases, and more. These already severe diseases are often exacerbated by an underlying and undetected celiac disease. Celiac disease that has not been diagnosed and remained untreated for decades dramatically increases the risk of otherwise rare small intestinal tumors and

© Springer Nature Switzerland AG 2019
D. Schuppan, K. Gisbert-Schuppan, *Wheat Syndromes*
https://doi.org/10.1007/978-3-030-19023-1_4

intestinal T cell lymphoma. These life-threatening complications, which are difficult to treat, are more than 100-fold more common in untreated celiacs than in the normal population.

With an estimated 80–90% of undiagnosed cases, the disease often goes undetected. This very high rate of undetected celiac disease can be explained—contrary to popular belief—by many cases that are not associated with classical symptoms, like abdominal pain or diarrhea.

The treatment of celiac disease consists of a strict gluten-free diet, i.e., the complete avoidance of products containing even traces of gluten. Naturally, patients have to completely abstain from the typical gluten-containing cereals wheat, barley, rye, spelt, emmer, and einkorn. For those affected, nutrition is complicated, since they have to avoid cereal products, such as bread and noodles, as well as processed foods. Most processed foods are enriched with gluten-containing cereals or purified gluten, and celiac disease can be triggered even by the smallest amounts of gluten. Only less than 20 mg/1000 g food is considered safe, and exclusively foods that fulfill this criterion can be declared as gluten free. The international seal for gluten-free products is the crossed-out ear of grain.

4.1.2   Epidemiology of Celiac Disease

Celiac disease is a common disease worldwide. Between 0.5 and 1.5% of the population are affected. This can reach 5% in some populations, as serological studies have shown. An exception is Southeast Asia, where celiac disease is rare due to a low prevalence of the genes HLA-DQ2/DQ8. There has been a dramatic increase of celiac disease cases in nomads from the Western Sahara who have been forced to settle in Algeria and have been living in camps for 40 years. These people have been flooded with wheat products in these camps, although cereals have traditionally not been part of their diet. More than 5% of the Saharaui population is now affected by celiac disease. Finland is another region where celiac disease is highly frequent with up to 2.5% of the elderly population. For a long time, celiac disease was believed to be rare in the US, but recent epidemiological studies, using the celiac blood test and confirmation by endoscopy, demonstrated an average prevalence of 1% as in most European and Mid-Eastern countries. Nevertheless, the number of unrecognized cases is very high and varies between 80% and 90% in most countries of the world, although celiac disease can now be clearly diagnosed with the tools and knowledge we have in the vast majority of patients.

With the high rate of undiagnosed cases, there is a need for a broader population screening, but due to high cost, its utility is still disputed among health care experts. In our view, heightened awareness and a lower threshold for diagnostic testing would be desirable. In general, it is recommended to screen close relatives of celiacs, patients with autoimmune diseases, and patients with some acute and chronic psychiatric and neurological disorders. In addition, celiac disease is a chameleon and may be suspected in patients with unexplained and diffuse diseases and symptoms. In view of the myriad symptoms, by which celiac disease can manifest, raising the awareness of general practitioners and specialists can significantly reduce the number of undetected cases. An example is Finland, where population screenings and increased awareness of high-risk patients and the manifold manifestations of celiac disease has significantly reduced the number of hidden cases. Here, the health system supports prevention and offers a comprehensive diagnostic system that has reduced the number of undetected celiacs to below 50%.

Generally, the prevalence of celiac disease has increased over the past 60 years. A study by the Mayo Clinic examined 50-year-old sera of military recruits using the blood test for transglutaminase antibodies to find a 4.5-fold lower prevalence than in a contemporary reference sample. This corresponded to a prevalence of 0.2% in the old sample and of 0.9% in the contemporary sample. There is still no plausible hypothesis to explain this difference since wheat consumption and gluten content has not changed significantly within these 50 years. It is likely that additional environmental factors and additional components in wheat (like ATI) are responsible for the high rate of celiac disease in today's populations.

4.1.3   History and Milestones of Celiac Disease Research

The first real breakthrough in the understanding of celiac disease was a discovery of the Dutch pediatrician Willem-Karel Dicke from Utrecht, The Netherlands, in the 1930s and 1940s. In the years of the German occupation during World War II, he discovered that children with severe abdominal pain, diarrhea, and pronounced malabsorption of nutrients improved once wheat products were not available due to food rationing. The unvoluntary wheat-free diet during these war times led to a drastic improvement in symptoms. Dicke had already made similar observations in the years before the war, when children with a failure to thrive recovered quickly on very restricted diets, such as a pure banana diet. After the war, Dicke conducted provocation experiments and found that the symptoms reoccurred rapidly when a wheat-containing diet was reintroduced. Together with the chemist van de Kamer, he was able to isolate gluten from the wheat as the detrimental component. Since then, celiac disease has also been called gluten-sensitive enteropathy. Gluten was also found in other related cereals such as rye and barley or early forms of wheat such as spelt, emmer, and einkorn. Following the introduction of the gluten-free diet, the acute mortality of affected children and adults fell from up to 30% to the level of the normal population. As a result, the then frequent clinical picture of children who despite a "normal" diet failed to thrive, had almost disappeared.

In the 1950s, the gluten-free diet was firmly established as an effective therapy for celiac disease. At this time, a novel diagnostic technology was developed to demonstrate the inflammatory reaction of the small intestine without having to resort to surgery. A small metal capsule that had to be swallowed was directed into the small intestine via a guidewire under X-ray control. Employing this minimally invasive device, duodenal tissue samples could be taken for histological examination. This method consistently showed villous atrophy and increased inflammatory cells as characteristic pathology and evidence of celiac disease. Until recently, the capsule has been used in children, as it can be performed without sedation. Since the 1970s, celiac disease has mainly been diagnosed using flexible endoscopy (see Sect. 4.1.6) that enables direct visualization of the small intestine and tissue sampling. In addition, a blood test for celiac disease, the so-called anti-endomysium antibody, was developed in the 1970s. However, it no longer plays a major role in diagnosis since the transglutaminase antibody test became available. The endomysium is the connective tissue that surrounds all smooth muscle cells, including those of the intestine. The enzyme transglutaminase is also found in the endomysium. The high prevalence of celiac disease among relatives already indicated a pronounced genetic predisposition. The key genetic markers for celiac disease were discovered in the early 1990s when the molecules HLA-DQ2 and HLA-DQ8 were identified as a necessary predisposition of the disease. The gene test for HLA-DQ2 and HLA-DQ8 currently plays an important role to rule out celiac disease in unclear cases.

In 1996, our group identified the autoantigen of celiac disease, tissue transglutaminase. An autoantigen is an endogenous molecule against which the body's own immune response is directed, in the case of celiac disease by producing autoantibodies (instead of triggering a T cell reaction). There are no relevant levels of such antibodies in healthy individuals. Autoantibodies are a specific feature of autoimmune diseases, i.e., diseases in which the body's immune system attacks the body's own cells or organs. The discovery of tissue transglutaminase as celiac disease autoantigen was another milestone. It helped to explain the pathogenesis of the disease better—as described below—and allowed to establish a serum test based on the detection of transglutaminase autoantibodies in the blood of patients. This test is now used worldwide to diagnose celiac disease noninvasively and to screen large populations for its prevalence. The antibodies are very useful to diagnose active celiac disease, but do not reflect well the level of the activity of the disease. We are currently developing an activity test that would permit to determine the extent of the inflammation in the small intestine. With such a blood test, it will be possible to immediately measure the response to the gluten-free diet and especially to novel therapies in celiac patients. Currently, the patients' intestinal response can only be quantified after several weeks of the gluten-free diet or a pharmacological intervention.

In summary, with the three identifiable factors leading to the disease—gluten, HLA-DQ2/HLA-DQ8, and transglutaminase—coeliac disease is one of the best understood (autoimmune) diseases (Fig. 4.1).

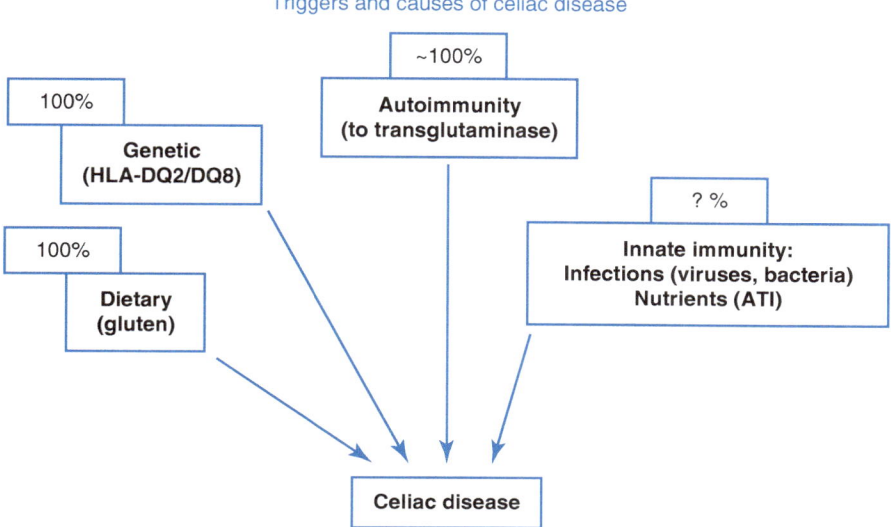

Fig. 4.1 Triggers of celiac disease. Celiac disease is the best understood intestinal immune disease. It is caused by a synergy between gluten, genetics and the auto-antigen transglutaminase (TG2). The reason why not all subjects that carry the key genetic predisposition, i.e., HLA-DQ2 or HLA-DQ8, develop celiac disease is mainly due to other environmental triggers, and only to a lesser degree caused by other genetic predispositions

4.1.4   Immunology of Celiac Disease

The digestion of bread and other cereal-foods already starts in the oral cavity where the salivary enzyme amylase begins to cleave starch into monosaccharides like glucose. Further digestion continues in the stomach through gastric acid and the protein-cleaving enzyme pepsin. Digestion takes up speed in the upper part of the small intestine (duodenum), where the gastric contents are neutralized, and pancreatic enzymes cleave almost all macromolecular carbohydrates, proteins, and lipids. Final cleavage into smallest molecules is carried out by enzymes on the surface of the intestinal epithelial cells. These smallest molecules are efficiently taken up as nutrients and transported by the bloodstream to the liver and other organs. However, a small proportion of uncleaved or incompletely cleaved food molecules reaches the lamina propria, the intestinal layer that carries most of the intestinal immune cells. The default setting of this immune-cell layer is to induce active tolerance against these food constituents, which are classified as friend. This usually also happens with the major protein of wheat, gluten. Gluten proteins are less completely digested by the human digestive enzymes than other food proteins. A significant fraction of these incompletely digested gluten peptides reaches the lamina propria. This leads to a relatively high concentration of gluten peptides of 10–40 amino acids length in the lamina propria in celiac as well as healthy subjects. Usually, these gluten peptides are sensed as being harmless by the intestinal immune system. However, in celiac patients, they are recognized as harmful, like an invading bug, and induce a rigorous defensive immune response, which causes collateral damage, with injury to the intestinal epithelial cells and tissue destruction, that finally results in villus atrophy.

Why does this self-destructive response to gluten occur only in celiac patients? Celiac patients have a genetic predisposition to recognize gluten peptides particularly well. The antigen-presenting cells in the gut of celiac patients are equipped with surface molecules that bind gluten peptides particularly well and present them to aggressive T cells. The T cells avidly grab the presented peptides via their receptors. This triggers the T cells' activation and proliferation, and now the inflammatory storm begins. The T cells multiply, release inflammatory substances, damage the epithelial cells and in the long run cause villus atrophy. Patients with celiac disease recognize the gluten peptides particularly well since their antigen presenting cells are equipped with special surface molecules. These are HLA-DQ2 and HLA-DQ8, the key genetic predisposition in people with celiac disease. Yet only 1% of the population develops celiac disease, although approximately one-third carry these genes. The abbreviation HLA stands for human leukocyte antigen and is due to the fact that these molecules were originally found on the surface of immune cells before their function for antigen presentation was recognized (see Fig. 4.2). It may take weeks, sometimes months or even years, until tissue destruction fully develops. Since the gluten-specific T cells that initially are present in only very few copies have multiplied thousands and millions of times, until the typical symptoms, such as reduced nutrient uptake, diarrhea or abdominal pain become manifest.

A particular breakthrough in understanding these relationships was a discovery made in our laboratory in 1996. We have shown that the body's own enzyme tissue transglutaminase that is produced in the intestinal mucosa reacts with the gluten peptides, forming complexes with them and altering their chemical nature. These changes induced by tissue transglutaminase allow the gluten peptides to be taken up more efficiently for improved presentation on the surface. This discovery was the prerequisite for a cascade of further important findings. For example, the research groups of Knut Lundin and Ludvig Sollid in Oslo, Norway, and Frits Koning in Leiden, The Netherlands, were able to independently demonstrate that transglutaminase can chemically alter the gluten peptides by changing their electrical charge from neutral to negative. Via this process of deamidation, the gluten peptides bind more firmly to HLA-DQ2 and HLA-DQ8. This causes a more vigorous T cell activation, indicating that the genetic predisposition can only fully come into play together with the autoantigen tissue transglutaminase (see Fig. 4.3). With the discovery of tissue transglutaminase as celiac disease autoantigen, it was shown for the first time that an auto-antigen is centrally involved in the pathogenesis of an (autoimmune) disease. For this reason, our discovery of tissue transglutaminase as celiac disease autoantigen is considered a paradigm shift not only in celiac disease research but also in the much broader field of immunology.

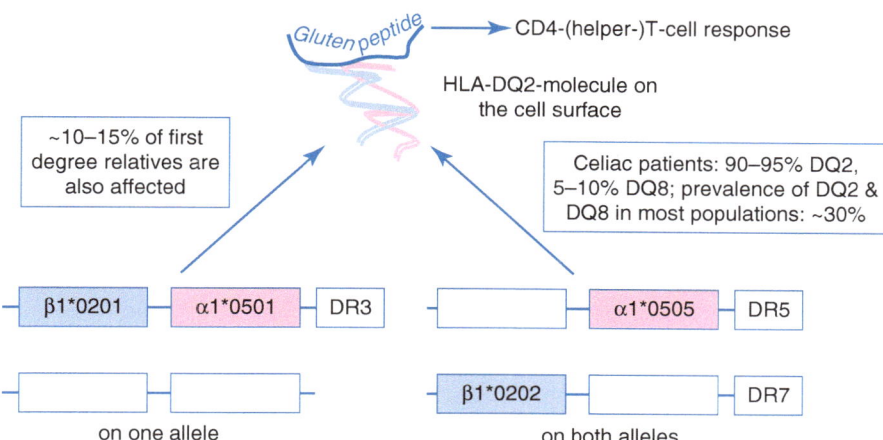

Fig. 4.2 Role of HLA-DQ2 in celiac disease. Each individual carries unique HLA (human leukocyte antigen)-proteins on his or her cells that consist of two protein chains. HLA class I molecules present microbial and tissue antigens and thus activate cytotoxic (CD8) T lymphocytes that kill virus-infected cells or cause rejection of another individual's cells or tissue after transplantation. HLA class II molecules present agents recognized as foreign, such as certain nutrient molecules, but also the body's self antigens in autoimmune diseases to (CD4) T lymphocytes. Only this interaction between HLA, antigen and the T cell leads to T cell activation and thus inflammation and tissue damage, or to active tolerance. In case of celiac disease, the HLA class II molecule DQ2 (or DQ8) that is mainly expressed on the surface of dendritic cells, macrophages an B lymphocytes recognizes and binds certain, incompletely digested gluten peptides of at least 11 amino acids length. Only when bound by HLA-DQ2 (or DQ8), the gluten peptides can trigger the activation of CD4 T lymphocytes. This means that there are no patients with celiac disease who are not carriers of HLA-DQ2 and/or -DQ8. On the other hand, between 30 and 50% of most populations have the DQ2- or DQ8-gene, but only one out of 30 of them will ever have celiac disease. The risk for celiac disease increases when subjects carry the double gene dose, i.e., each of their diploid (duplicated) chromosomes expresses the two HLA-DQ2 (or DQ8) protein chains, instead of a single gene copy on one of the chromosomes. The occurrence of DQ2 and DQ8 is associated with another set of HLA-genes, DR3 and DR4, respectively. These can bind other self-antigens and are therefore central preconditions for various autoimmune diseases, largely explaining the high rate of autoimmune diseases in patients with celiac disease

T cell proliferation, as well as the release of inflammatory substances, are only activated for as long as gluten is ingested and subside when gluten is not further supplied. When gluten is consumed, the lymphocytes react like gluten was an intruder. In a microbial infection, the T cells would finally get control over and eliminate the invader. In contrast, in celiac disease, there is a continuous flow of gluten peptides that cannot be reduced by the T cells and causes their ongoing activation. Therefore, it is no wonder that in untreated celiac disease, severe damage occurs that eventually culminates in an architectural remodeling and loss of the villi, that are needed to resorb the nutrients. This also explains the known complications of malabsorption in celiac patients, since the nutrients can only be absorbed via the huge intestinal surface that is formed by the villus' finger-like protrusions. Once the villi have disappeared, the intestinal surface is dramatically reduced. Moreover, the

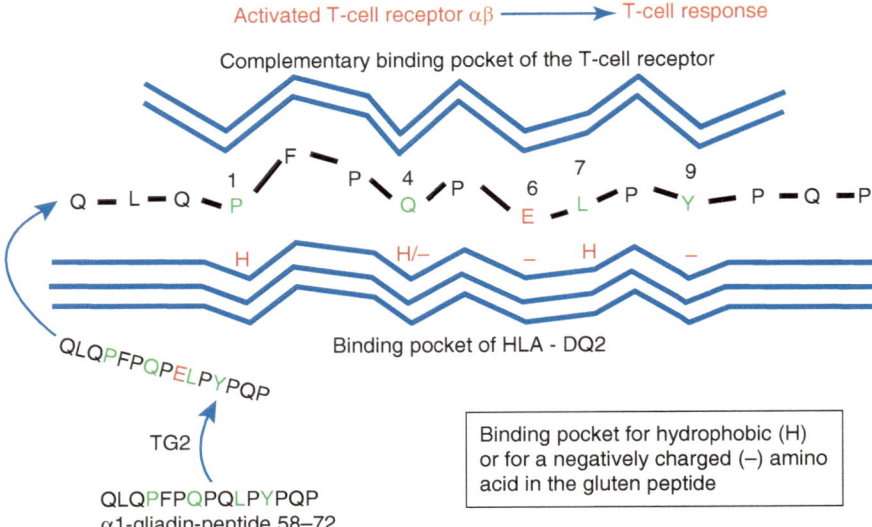

Fig. 4.3 Immune activation by transglutaminase and gluten. The 15 amino acids long gliadin peptide α1(58–72) remains undigested, is partly resobed by the intestinal mucosa and reaches the lamina propria, i.e., the immune cell layer underneath the intestinal epithelium. There it encounters the enzyme transglutaminase (TG2) that converts one of its glutamine residues (Q, neutral charge) to a glutamic acid residue (E, negatively charged). With this change of charge, the resultant gliadin peptide now fits much better into the antigen binding pocket of the HLA-DQ2 molecule on the antigen presenting cells. This binding pocket specifically recognizes 5 of the 9 embedded amino acids of the gliadin peptide (color coded) and requires the negatively charged glutamic acid that was just generated by the reaction with TG2. Only now the gliadin specific T cell can recognize the gluten peptide and gets activated. (amino acids described by the one letter code: *Q* glutamine, *L* leucine, *P* proline, *F* phenylalanine, *E* glutamic acid, *Y* tyrosine)

inflammatory T cells cause direct damage to the epithelial cells that leads to their loss of function and premature shedding into the lumen. The gut reacts to the enhanced epithelial cell turnover by activating its intestinal stem cell compartment, the so-called crypts. The crypts are indentations that alternate with the villous protrusions. Therefore, another histological hallmark of celiac disease is the deepening of these indentations, called crypt hyperplasia.

The nutritional gluten fuels the small intestinal inflammation. Once the fuel is cut off by a strict gluten-free diet, the inflammation subsides, and the mucosa starts to regenerate. Full regeneration can take months to years, although most patients report a significant symptomatic improvement after 2 weeks on the gluten-free diet. The immunological processes are illustrated in Fig. 4.4. Why does only 1 person out of 30 carriers of HLA-DQ2 or HLA-DQ8 develop celiac disease in his/her lifetime? This has not yet been clarified in detail. Contributing factors are disturbances in immune regulation by other genes that are less relevant than HLA-DQ2 and HLA-DQ8. Likely more important are nutritional factors in early childhood, acute intestinal infections, oral medications, environmental chemicals, and repeated antibiotic therapies that

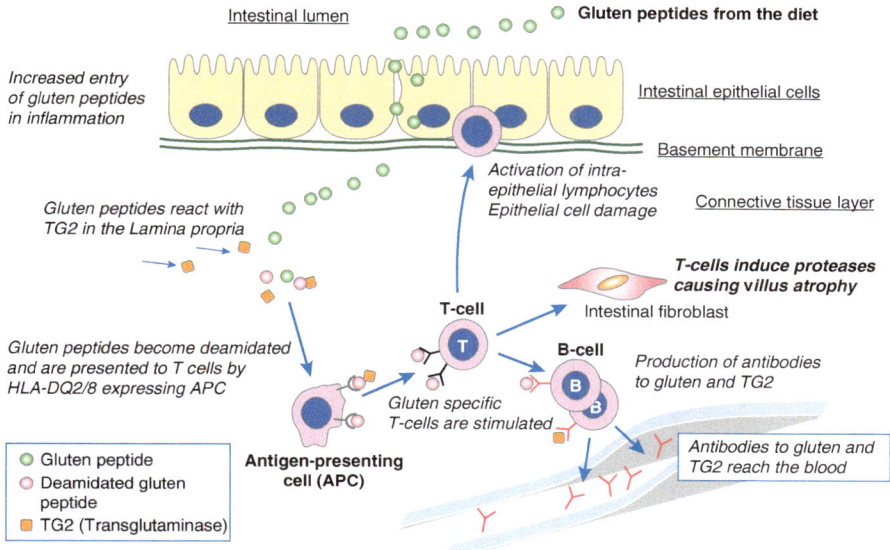

Fig. 4.4 Immunology of celiac disease. Undigested immunogenic gluten peptides reach the lamina propria underneath the intestinal epithelial cells. This uptake is promoted by factors that increase the permeability of the intestinal epithelial cell layer, such as gut infections or certain medications, but also by an increased active uptake by and transport through the epithelial cells. In the lamina propria they are (chemically) modified by the enzyme transglutaminase (TG2) that is upregulated in different intestinal cells during inflammation. Specifically, TG2 deamidates these gluten peptides, as described in the previous figure, which changes the peptides'charge from neutral to negatively charged. This change in charge enables them to bind efficiently to the surface molecules HLA-DQ2 or -DQ8 on the antigen-presenting cells (APC), mainly dendritic cells, macrophages and B lymphocytes. Moreover, TG2 forms larger complexes with these gluten peptides that are preferentially ingested (phagocytosed), processed and then presented by the APC. The peptide that is presented via HLA-DQ2 or HLA-DQ8 can now activate T-lymphocytes, even if these are present in low quantities, that carry a receptor for just this gluten peptide (key and lock principle). What follows is a several 1000-fold multiplication of this T lymphocyte clone by cell division over the following days and weeks. Similar multiplications occur for other gluten peptides and their respective T lymphocyte clones. The activated T cells secrete cytokines and chemokines (messenger proteins) that initiate and sustain the proliferation of B lymphocytes that also carry, slightly different, preformed receptors for each gluten peptide, including the peptides deamidated by TG2, or even for TG2 itself. Therefore, these B lymphocytes produce the circulating antibodies that are the basis for the serological diagnosis of celiac disease. The activated immune cells also release cytokines and chemokines that attract and activate other immune and non-immune cells, e.g., macrophages and fibroblasts that secrete tissue destructive enzymes and thereby destroy the intestinal architecture. A minor amount of the gluten peptides can also be presented on the surface of the intestinal epithelial cells that also possess HLA-molecules, or lead to the expression of danger molecules on their surface. These danger molecules serve as alarm signals for killer or cytotoxic T cells that can attack and even destroy the epithelia, similar to the elimination of virus-infected cells. All these inflammatory pathways contribute to villous atrophy, crypt hyperplasia, and epithelial cell damage, the histological hallmarks of celiac disease, often leading to malabsorption, the sequela of chronic nutrient deficiency, and occasionally intestinal cancer

affect the intestinal microbiota. Such influences can negatively affect the immune system that is primed for tolerance, including tolerance to gluten. These hypotheses also help to explain why nowadays at least 50% of celiac disease cases are diagnosed in adults, who often present with previously unexperienced symptoms.

4.1.5 Manifestations of Celiac Disease

Although celiac disease is an inflammatory disease that is located predominantly in the small intestine, its symptoms are not necessarily related to the gastrointestinal tract and digestion. Not only patients but also doctors are often surprised when they learn that the typical symptoms are not abdominal pain, bloating, or diarrhea. Rather, the symptoms show an astonishing range and therefore often are not attributed to celiac disease. In this regard, the majority of adult patients does not experience the "classical" abdominal symptoms (see Fig. 4.5). For this reason, celiac disease has been dubbed the "chameleon of internal medicine".

The course of disease is different in infants and young children. In fact, most of the very young patients suffer from classical symptoms that more quickly raise the suspicion of celiac disease. These are diarrhea, abdominal pain and bloating as well

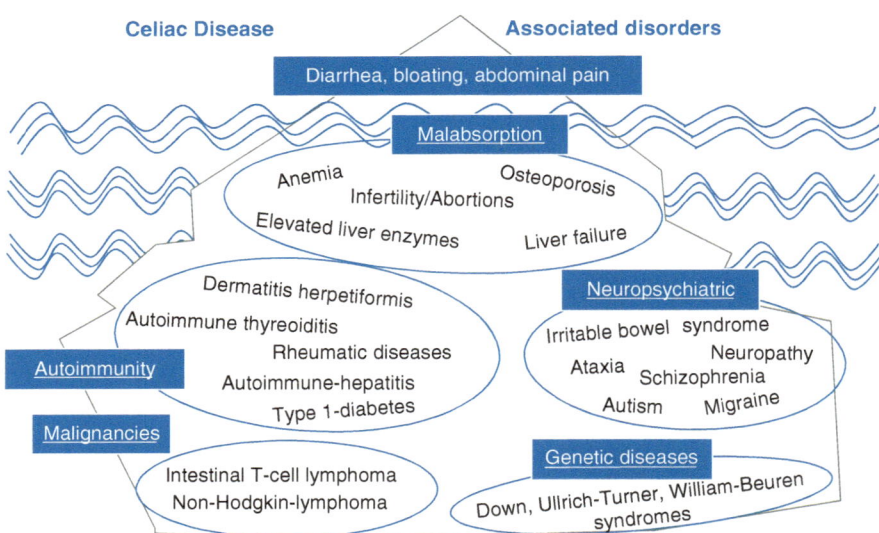

Fig. 4.5 Diseases that are associated with celiac disease. The classical symptoms of celiac disease, with diarrhea, bloating and abdominal pain represent only the tip of the celiac iceberg. Most of the patients do not have these complaints, or only minor symptoms. The spectrum of associated diseases comprises sequelae of malabsorption of nutrients and vitamins, several autoimmune diseases, certian cancers and otherwise unexplained neurological and psychiatric diseases. Moreover, some genetic diseases with chromosomal aberrations are linked to celiac disease

as underweight and failure to thrive, but also crankiness and whininess. Special attention should always be paid to children from celiac families. We recommend to test them routinely for celiac disease, even when they appear healthy. Prominent symptoms of children and adults with celiac disease are summarized in Table 4.1.

In adults, the disease is often discovered rather by chance due to unspecific symptoms. However, as soon as they are on the gluten-free diet, these patients quickly feel much better and notice that they have previously been unwell. Usually, these patients have mild and unspecific symptoms of the disease, such as fatigue and some abdominal discomfort. The second group of patients becomes symptomatic in adulthood, but with acute onset and severe symptoms, including profuse diarrhea, attacks of abdominal pain, or a sudden decline in performance and wellbeing. These patients may have had a low-level celiac disease before that became manifest after another trigger. Typical triggers are bacterial or viral infections or a long-lasting antibiotic treatment causing dysbiosis, i.e., an unfavorable change of the intestinal microbiota. These patients may have had a long-lasting low-level celiac disease before that went unnoticed. The third group of patients presents with signs of malabsorption, i.e., a deficiency of vitamins, trace elements and sometimes protein stores, and often with anemia. Such deficiencies are often detected by chance when routine blood work is done in patients who complain of unspecific symptoms. A fourth and last group are patients with autoimmune diseases. Prominently in adults,

Table 4.1 Symptoms of celiac disease

Classical	Children/adolescents (n = 251)	Adults (n = 359)
	Frequency	
Diarrhea	28 – 55%	18 – 47%
Abdominal pain	12 – 33%	18 – 28%
Severe bloating/ extended abdomen	12 – 29%	26%
Anemia	2 – 19%	38 – 51%
Weight loss/ weight below 5th percentile	13 – 26%	34%
Growth retardation	9 – 16%	--

Atypical	
	Dental enamel defects
Chronic fatigue/ reduced performance	Selective IgA deficiency
Difficulty to concentrate	Recurrent apthous stomatitis
Depressed mood	
Chronische constipation	Unclear elevation of liver enzymes
	Fatty liver
Retarded puperty (Amenorrhea)	Cardiomyopathy
Infertility (women and men)	
	Chronic headaches/ migraine
Iron deficiency anemia	Polyneuropathy
Osteoporosis/ osteopenia	Ataxia
	Epilepsy

Frequencies of symptoms in newly diagnosed patients on a gluten containing diet celiac disease is an indicator for (other) autoimmune diseases, but also vice versa, patients with autoimmune diseases often suffer from celiac disease.

This raises the question if celiac disease itself should be classified as an autoimmune disease. On the one hand, celiac disease shows the characteristics of an autoimmune disease, especially autoantibodies against tissue transglutaminase. On the other hand, the disease is usually cured with the strictly gluten-free diet, and gluten is not the body's own structure. In typical autoimmune diseases, that are characterized by autoantibodies against the body's own structures, there is no identified trigger that can be excluded. Since celiac disease shows features of an autoimmune disease, i.e., autoantibodies against tissue transglutaminase, celiac disease may be described as a "partial autoimmune disease".

However, celiac disease is highly associated with classical autoimmune diseases. Several studies have shown that on average 30% of adult celiac patients are affected by one or more of the following autoimmune diseases: Insulin deficient type 1 diabetes, autoimmune thyroid diseases like as Hashimoto's thyroiditis or Graves' disease, rheumatic diseases such as rheumatoid arthritis, scleroderma, Behcet's disease, blistering dermatitis herpetiformis, or autoimmune liver diseases and several more (see Table 4.2).

Table 4.2 Celiac disease associated diseases

Autoimmune diseases	Prevalence in celiac disease
Autoimmune thyreoiditis	3 – 7%
Autoimmune hepatitis (children)	12 – 13%
Autoimmune hepatitis (adults)	2 – 3%
Diabetes mellitus type 1	2 – 12%
Dermatitis herpetiformis	2 – 4%
Juvenile polyarthritis	1.5 – 2.5%
Psoriasis	
Autoimmune alopecia	
Sjoegren's syndrome	
Atrophic gastritis	
Vasculitis/ collagen diseases	
Addison' disease	
Genetic diseases	
Down syndrome	5 – 12%
Ullrich-Turner syndrome	2 – 5%
Williams-Beuren syndrome	9%

Prevalence—percentage of celiac disease patients with this condition; this is increased severalfold compared to the general population; percentages taken from several studies

The prevalence of autoimmune diseases is lower in celiac children, but still far above population controls. It is still controversial how far the gluten-free diet may also prevent or improve the associated autoimmune diseases. Improvement is certainly not possible for patients with manifest type 1 diabetes or advanced thyroid dysfunction, where damage to the pancreas or the thyroid gland has led to a complete loss of function. Less information is available for prevention of these or other autoimmune diseases. In young children from high-risk families, i.e., families in which at least one parent has celiac disease or type 1 diabetes, an early gluten-free diet may prevent or at least delay the onset of autoimmunity. Large prospective studies addressing these questions are currently being performed in several clinical centers worldwide.

4.1.6 How to Detect Celiac Disease?

When celiac disease is suspected, and the patient is still consuming gluten or has consumed gluten until recently, not more than a few weeks ago, diagnosis is straight-forward. The vast majority of these patients has elevated blood levels of antibodies against tissue transglutaminase that are usually increased two to tenfold above normal. Even if patients have already started a gluten-free diet, increased antibody levels can be detected for weeks or months, depending on the initial titer. The reason for the prolonged detectability of the autoantibodies is that their half-life, i.e., the time until the antibodies have dropped back to half of their initial value, is approximately 40–60 days. For example a patient with a fivefold increased antibody titer may need up to half a year on a gluten-free diet until the autoantibodies have reached the normal range.

In case of a positive antibody test, an endoscopy with sampling from the small intestine is usually performed for confirmation. This sounds frightening for many patients but is actually a minimally invasive procedure with a very low risk. The procedure takes 5–10 min, is performed under mild sedation and does not cause pain. Sedation means that the patients receive mild general anesthesia, i.e., they are responsive but usually do not remember the examination later. The endoscope is inserted into the upper small intestine through the mouth, esophagus, and stomach. It consists of a flexible rubber-coated controllable tube of 130 cm (51 inches) length and harbors several channels. These channels contain:

- the power cable for a light source,
- a fiber-optic cable for receiving the image that is transmitted directly to a large screen in high resolution,
- a tube through which air can be supplied to mildly inflate the stomach and intestine for better visibility or by which fluid can be removed,
- and finally, a channel through which water rinsing of mucus or blood can be performed and which also serves as channel for the biopsy forceps that allows taking tissue sampling.

At the endoscope's tip are the strong light source and the camera that enables the endoscopist to see all the details of the esophagus, stomach, and upper small intestine on the screen. The examiner can then introduce the biopsy forceps, which is located on the tip of a long wire, into the biopsy channel under direct vision. Inspection of the upper small intestine (duodenum) is particularly important since here the inflammatory lesions of celiac disease are found. The endoscopist can now take several targeted biopsies. To this aim, he can insert the forceps, take the biopsy, which is pulled back through the endoscope, deposit it in a container, and reinsert the forceps for the next biopsy. This does not require to take out the endoscope after each biopsy. The biopsy samples are tiny, measuring of 3–4 mm (0.12–0.16 inches) and do not inflict any significant damage to the mucosa. Upper endoscopy and biopsy sampling is one of the safest procedures in gastroenterology (Figs. 4.6 and 4.7).

The expert guidelines for celiac disease demand at least four biopsies to be taken from the upper part of the small intestine for histological examination by the expert pathologist. The pathological examination requires preparation of 5 μm thin sections of the samples and their staining with special dyes to visualize tissue architecture and the cells. This allows a standardized assessed of inflammation and villus atrophy (Fig. 4.8). When villus atrophy is found, the diagnosis of celiac disease is confirmed and the degree of damage according to the Marsh classification determined (Fig. 4.9). To obtain the result normally takes one to 3 days. It is not uncommon that inflammatory changes are described that are not typical for celiac disease. In these cases, the expert has to decide if these uncharacteristic findings are compatible with the diagnosis of celiac disease. In such ambiguous cases, the genetic test for HLA-DQ2 and HLA-DQ8 can be useful. If this test is negative, celiac disease

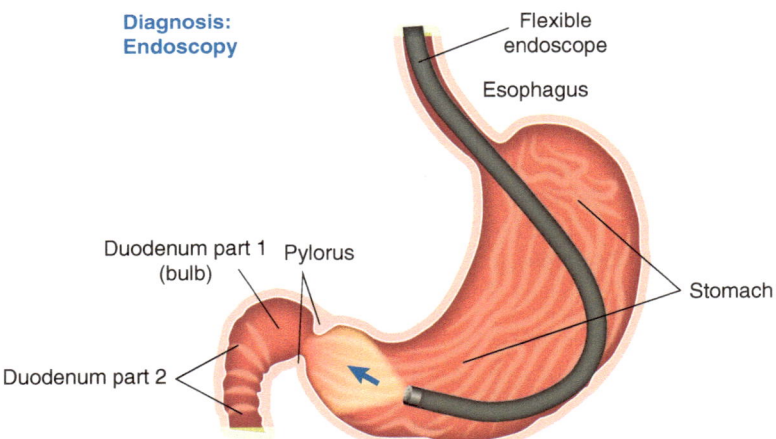

Fig. 4.6 Endoscopic diagnosis (1). The flexible endoscope is introduced under vision via the oral cavity and the esophagus into the stomach and upper small intestine. The endoscope allows biopsy sampling from all parts of the esophagus, stomach and upper small intestine, in celiac disease primarily from the second part of the duodenum

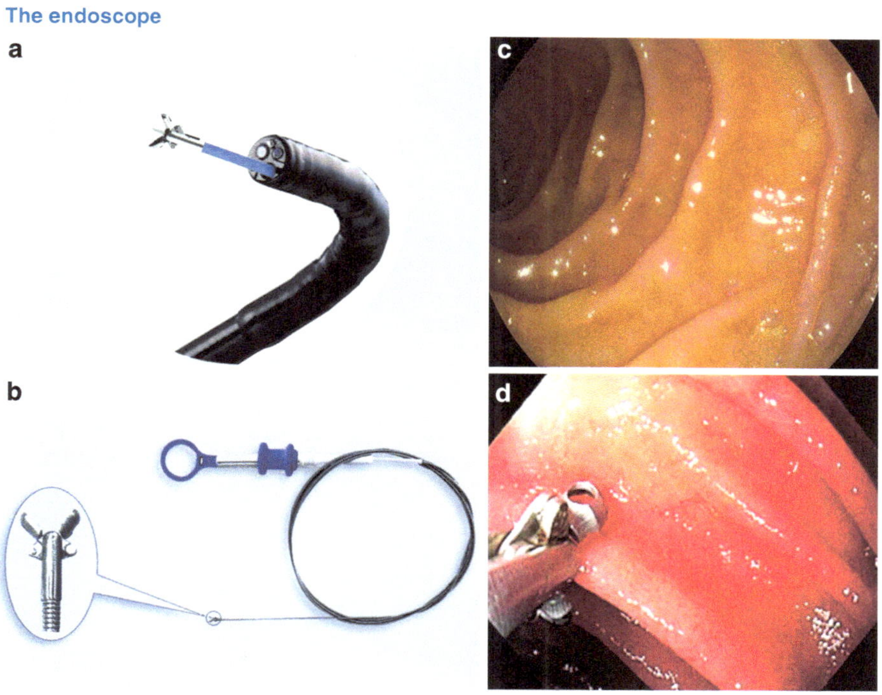

The endoscope

Fig. 4.7 **Endoscopic diagnosis (2)**. (**a**) The endoscope is equipped with a fiberoptic cable for the light source, one fiberoptic cable or a cable with a sensor chip for the real time camera, a channel for flushing with water and supply of air (to rinse and mildly inflate the organs for better visibility) and a channel to introduce the flexible biopsy forceps attached to a long wire and to be operated by an assistant from the examiner side of the endoscope (here the forceps is opened). (**b**) The biopsy forceps is opened or closed by the assistant via a handle outside of the endoscope. (**c**) Normal mucosa and mucosal folds of the second part of the duodenum. (**d**) Opened biopsy forceps. A tissue sample of approx. 0.3 cm (1/8 in.) is taken. The closed biopsy forceps with the sample is withdrawn through the endoscope channel by the assistant, and asservated in fixative for histological examination

can be excluded. In case of a positive finding, celiac disease is possible but not proven, since one-third of the population are carriers of HLA-DQ2 and/or HLA-DQ8 without ever developing the disease. The genetic test can be performed in a blood sample but is currently only available in special laboratories.

However, in real life we have to consider differential diagnosis to celiac disease. We see many patients who live gluten-free for a long time without ever having been diagnosed with celiac disease, but who after many years of a gluten-free diet want to have a clear diagnosis. Mostly, these are patients who are convinced that they are better off on a gluten-free diet and who have experienced that they develop symptoms after eating gluten-containing foods. One may ask, why it should be important to diagnose celiac disease if patients eat gluten-free anyway and feel better that way? A clear diagnosis is indeed important because patients with celiac

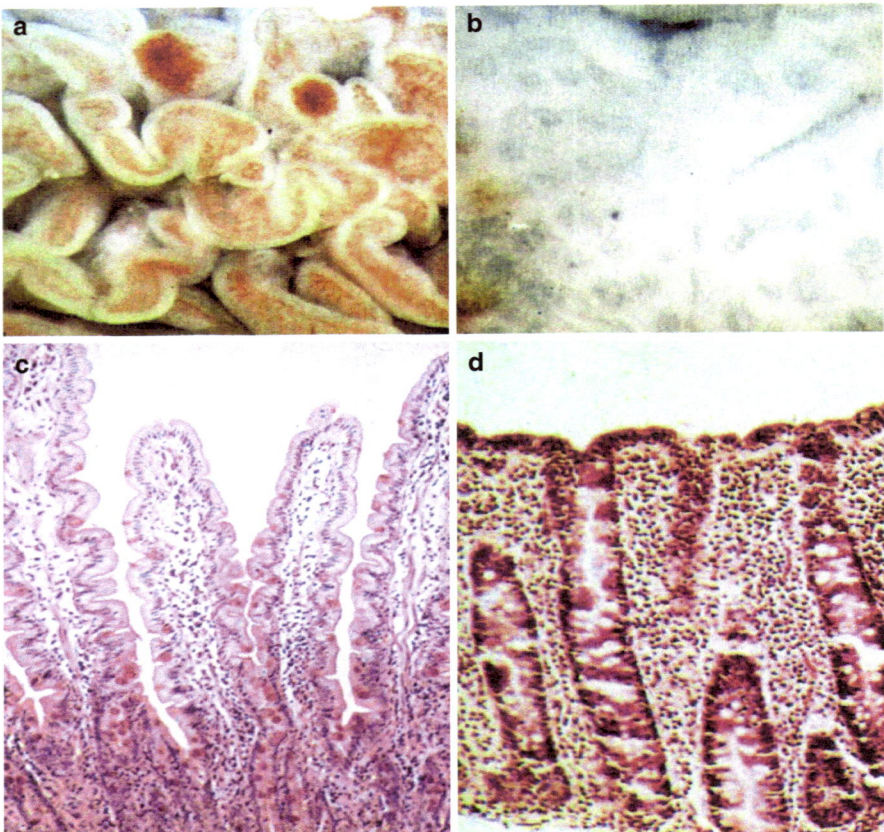

Fig. 4.8 Histological diagnosis. Microscopy of a freshly taken intestinal biopsy: (**a**) normal duodenal villi; (**b**) complete villous atrophy in celiac disease. (**c, d**) Histological correlates of **a** and **b** after fixation and embedding of the biopsy, slicing and staining of thin tissue sections

disease must follow the strict gluten-free diet. Celiac patients have to stay away not only from obvious gluten-containing foods, such as bread, pizza, pasta, cakes, and biscuits but also have to avoid any foods that may contain hidden, tiny amounts of gluten, as are usually found in prepared foods, such as sauces, sweets, spices and many more. If, on the other hand, patients have an ATI-sensitivity, as detailed in Chap. 5, and therefore feel better when not consuming gluten-containing foods, not the strict, but only a largely gluten-free diet is required. This means only a reduction of gluten-containing foods by 90–95%. i.e., only evident sources of gluten need to be avoided. The reason for this is that gluten-containing foods are always ATI-containing foods. Thus, there is no need to pay too much attention to possible hidden sources of gluten for patients with ATI-sensitivity. Another differential diagnosis that needs to be considered is typical or atypical wheat allergy that we introduce and discuss in Chap. 7.

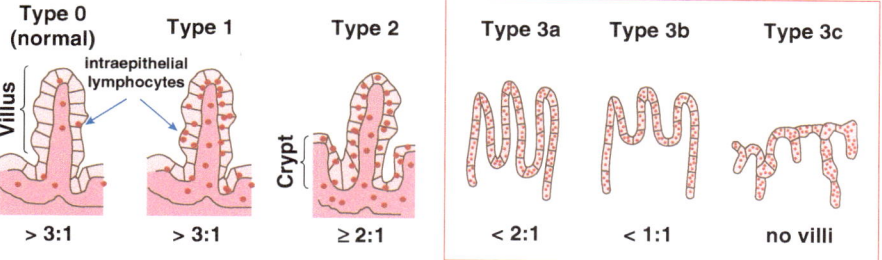

Ratio villus height : Crypt depth

Fig. 4.9 Histological classification of celiac disease. Tissue samples are taken from the duodenum during upper endoscopy using a small biopsy forceps. Samples are fixed, embedded, sectioned and stained for microscopical examination by a pathologist. Biopsies are generally assessed according to the Marsh and Oberhuber classification. Type 0: normal mucosa, ratio of villus height to crypt depth above 3:1, normal numbers of immune cells (mostly lymphocytes); Type 1: increased numbers of intraepithelial lymphocytes (IEL, located within the epithelial cell layer; more than 25 per 100 epithelial cells); this finding is not specific for celiac disease—in about 85% of cases increased IEL are indicative of patients with food allergy or infections; Type 2: as in type I, but with deepened crypts, rare, but more specific for celiac disease; Type 3: partial, subtotal or total villus atrophy, always combined with crypt hyperplasia; specific for celiac disease once other, rare causes have been ruled out, especially when serum autoantibodies to TG2 are elevated; the Marsh 3b lesion (subtotal villus atrophy), is most frequently found in active celiac disease

4.1.7   Treatment of Celiac Disease

Regarding treatment, the bad news is: Apart from a strictly gluten-free diet, to date, there is no effective alternative therapy for celiac patients. However, the good news is that several research groups and drug companies are working on different pharmacological therapies.

We present these pharmacological approaches in more detail below because patients are highly interested in alternative therapies, and we are regularly asked about therapy options in our consultations as well as in public lectures. Indeed, celiac patients were greatly helped if a drug was available that would alleviate their sensitivity to gluten. However, currently, it is unlikely that a drug will ever allow safe, unlimited consumption of gluten. It is more realistic that such therapy will eliminate the necessity of the strict gluten-free diet, meaning that patients will not have to pay too much attention to hidden gluten. This alone will significantly improve the patients' quality of life since in their experience the largest psychological and social burden is not having to avoid the obvious sources but to live in fear of hidden gluten. This, even more, applies to patients with refractory coeliac disease type 1 who already react to the smallest amounts of gluten.

Set aside these difficulties, the gluten-free diet, in general, is difficult for many reasons. Patients frequently state that it is unpleasant for them to live without the

Where gluten is found

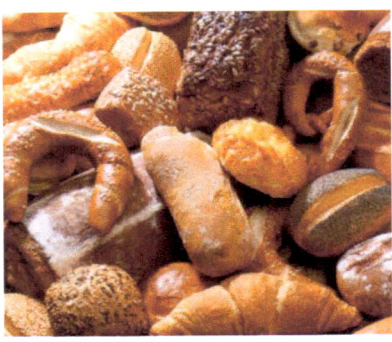

• Beer	• Rice syrup
• Broths	• Salat dressings
• Flavor additives	• Soft drinks
• Spices	• Starch
• Yeast	• Sweets
• Licorice	• Tea preparations
• Malt vinegar	• nearly all refined foods...
• Medications	

Fig. 4.10 Foods that contain gluten. Gluten can be found in most refined foods

Fig. 4.11 Gluten content in pasta and bread. Highly reactive (sensitive) celiac patients can develop intestinal inflammation with as little as 50 mg gluten per day

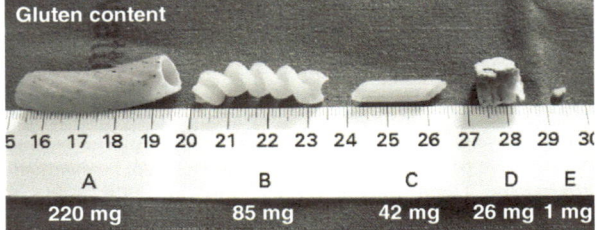

special taste and sensory qualities of gluten-containing products. They miss crispy rolls and pizza, pasta al dente, and soft and airy cakes and biscuits, and they are often not satisfied with alternative products. At least, alternative products have now become increasingly common and broadly available. It is also particularly problematic to adhere to the strict diet when patients eat out, because even if a meal is declared gluten-free, it may contain significant amounts of gluten, especially when a kitchen is not maintained gluten-free. Gluten is also found in almost all refined foods and food additives (Fig. 4.10). Some celiac patients can tolerate minor amounts of gluten, but others are highly sensitive and react with symptoms. A study from Italy shows that 10–50 mg of gluten daily—a normal daily consumption is between 10 and 20 g per day—can lead to small intestinal damage within 2 weeks. 10 mg is equivalent to a quarter of a small spaghetti noodle (Fig. 4.11).

Therefore, celiac patients would be greatly helped if there were a drug that could eliminate the effect of small amounts of gluten in food. Researchers, biotech, and pharmaceutical companies have developed therapeutic strategies that may be able to neutralize these smaller amounts of gluten. In the following, we highlight 4 major approaches:

1. Gluten-degrading enzymes are a much-discussed strategy to destroy the immunogenic gluten peptides in the food before they reach the duodenum and can activate the intestinal immune system. A promising pilot study in 41 selected celiac patients was performed who were in complete remission on a longer gluten-free diet, showing no symptoms, no intestinal lesions, and no autoantibodies.

They received a daily 3 g of gluten mixed into orange juice for 6 weeks. One group received the drink with, the other group without the gluten-degrading enzymes (a mix of a microbial and a germinating barley enzyme). In this study, the enzymes were able to prevent intestinal damage. A follow-up study was then conducted in 500 patients who, despite a strictly gluten-free diet (i.e., suspected refractory celiac disease type 1), were still suffering from intestinal damage and frequent complaints. They received either a placebo or the enzymes for 12–24 weeks. Here the enzyme therapy was disappointing because the inflammatory activity did not improve compared to the placebo-treated patients, and the symptoms even tended to increase. How can this be explained? In the first, successful study, patients received the enzymes together with a suspension of gluten, creating optimal conditions for complete degradation of the gluten peptides. In the second study, which included patients with high sensitivity towards minimal amounts of gluten (because they still had intestinal damage despite their strict gluten-free diet), the enzymes had to be extremely active, to completely digest the gluten in the complex ingested food, before it reaches the duodenum. This requires not only their complete mixing with the food mash in the stomach in a short time but also a long-lasting enzyme activity that is not inhibited by other food components. Obviously, in this second study and under real-life conditions, the enzymes were not active enough to completely deactivate the gluten. Only the second study represents the real-life scenario that celiac patients encounter. This is a general problem of enzyme therapies. However, another study is planned that employs a synthetic enzyme with 100-fold higher activity against gluten, the so-called Kuma Protease. It will be interesting to see if this novel enzyme will meet the challenge of real-life gluten ingestion.

2. A second approach is based on findings that cholera bacteria release a toxin, the so-called ZOT (zonula occludens toxin), that opens the tight junctions between the intestinal epithelial cells. This toxin causes profuse diarrhea in patients with cholera. The damaged intestinal epithelial cells release a protein, called zonulin, that exerts a similar effect. Excess zonulin is also increasingly produced in celiac disease. A small synthetic peptide called Larazotide is supposed to block the effect of zonulin on a postulated but never identified epithelial cell receptor. Thus, Larazotide would reconstitute the tight junctions and re-establish an intact intestinal barrier. More than 1000 patients have been treated with Larazotide in several studies that have produced different results. In none of these studies, a histological assessment was performed to confirm an improvement of the intestinal inflammation that is the main criterion for efficacy, as defined by the regulatory authorities. In some studies, patients showed only a subjective improvement, unexpectedly at the lowest in contrast to the highest dose of the drug. Due to the counterintuitive results, studies on this approach have been abandoned for a while. However, recently, a large clinical study in patients with residual celiac disease activity has been initiated based on novel mechanistic ideas to explain the efficacy of the low dose of the drug. The idea behind this is that higher doses activate counter-regulatory mechanisms.

3. A third strategy is the so-called gluten vaccination. The rationale derives from well conducted preclinical studies that have shown that about 60% of celiac patients show a strong T cell reaction against three gluten peptides from wheat

and rye. The underlying hypothesis is similar to hypo-sensitization in allergies, where the allergen is injected or ingested in small but increasing doses to induce tolerance to the allergen. Gluten vaccination is supposed to work the same way. The three predominant gluten peptides should generate tolerance to gluten in celiac patients. To date, more than 100 patients have been tested with the gluten vaccine. These so-called phase 1 studies showed that subjects developed some cytokine and T cell patterns in the blood that may indicate the potential of tolerance development. However, a gluten-challenge study in a larger number of patients is still pending. One problem is that the immune mechanism underlying celiac disease does not resemble an allergy. In allergies, hypo-sensitization induces allergen-blocking IgG antibodies, whereas in celiac disease we are dealing with a T cell reaction in which the blocking of gluten by antibodies plays virtually no role. Experts are still waiting for the larger phase 2 clinical study, originally announced for 2017, in which a large number of patients with gluten provocations will be tested for the prophylactic effect of this vaccination.

4. The fourth, and in our opinion the most promising approach, is the specific inhibition of tissue transglutaminase, the enzyme that makes gluten peptides immunogenic and thereby promotes the inflammation, using a small molecular drug that can be taken as a pill. A phase 1 clinical study involving more than 100 subjects has demonstrated the drug's good tolerability and bioavailability. A phase 2 clinical study in 160 patients has started in the summer of 2018. This approach seems to be the most promising, as the drug is absorbed by the intestinal mucosa, to inhibit the activity of intestinal tissue transglutaminase over a prolonged period of time. This should lead to a longer-lasting intestinal protection since the drug prevents deamidation and thus immunological potentiation of the gluten peptides by transglutaminase. This treatment should be effective, even in the presence of immunogenic gluten peptides in the intestinal lumen. The aim of such therapy would be to alleviate the extremely strict gluten-free diet of celiac patients that is much more difficult than simply to avoid evidently gluten-containing foods. Especially, patients with refractory celiac disease type 1, who are extremely sensitive to micro-quantities of gluten, could benefit greatly from this therapy when used as a supportive medication. The four major and other pharmacological approaches are illustrated in Fig. 4.12.

4.1.8   Summary

To sum up, celiac disease is a serious inflammatory disease that is originating in the small intestine and caused by nutritional gluten. The intestinal immune system in these patients senses gluten as if it were a dangerous invader, such as certain viruses or bacteria. This triggers intestinal inflammation and can also lead to manifold symptoms outside of the gut. The variety of symptoms, that often are not abdominal complaints, is one reason why up to 90% of patients remain undetected. After diagnosis, patients must follow the strict gluten-free diet. The

New therapeutic approaches for celiac disease

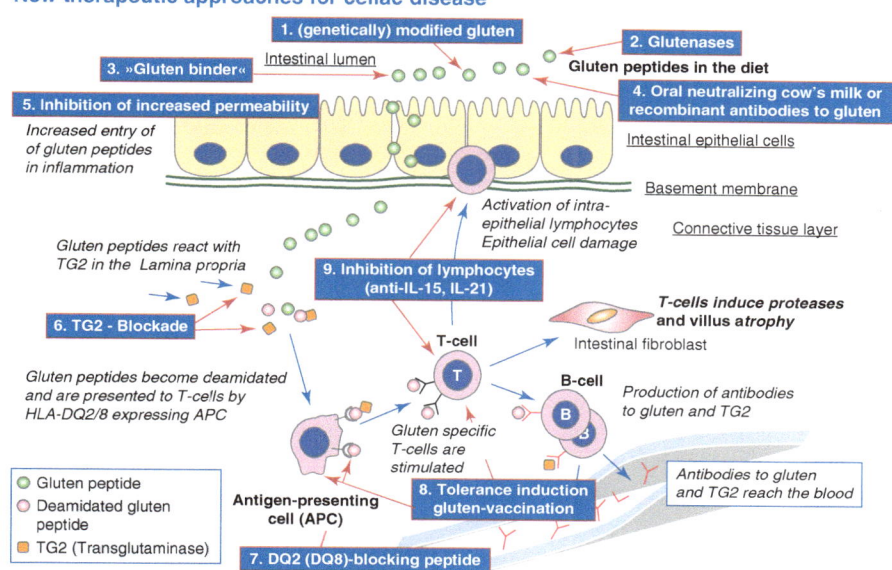

Fig. 4.12   Novel therapies for celiac disease. Pharmacological therapies aim at neutralization of minor to modest amounts of gluten in the food (not more than 3 g daily in view of 15–20 g average consumption with a normal diet). Promising approaches are glutenases (gluten degrading enzymes, 2), and inhibitors of TG2 (7). The possibility to reach a state of tolerance to ingested gluten by a prophylactic subcutaneous vaccination with immunogenic gluten peptides (8) would possibly provide a cure, but its rationale and potential efficacy is discussed controversially. Immunosuppressive drugs like antibodies that, e.g., block the pro-inflammatory cytokine interleukin (IL)-15 (9) are currently tested in patients with refractory celiac disease

diagnosis of active celiac disease is relatively straightforward, but there are unclear cases that need to be assessed by a specialist. In addition to celiac disease, there are other inflammatory diseases caused by gluten-containing foods: The classical and the atypical wheat allergies as well as ATI sensitivity. These need to be differentiated from celiac disease.

4.2   Case Vignettes: Celiac Disease

4.2.1   Patient Thomas H. (48 Years): Celiac Disease after Food Poisoning

Thomas H. is a patient in whom the symptoms of celiac disease were not apparent until adulthood. He is 48 years old and has always been healthy except for some childhood illnesses. During a vacation in Mexico, he suffers from acute diarrhea with vomiting that he attributes to "food poisoning" by a shellfish dish. After 1 week, already back home, the acute symptoms improve, but he still complains of abdominal pain and diarrhea. Over the next 2 months he experiences a persistent loss of appetite, mild nausea, and loses 18 lb of weight. His primary care physician arranges for a stool test for pathogenic bacteria, parasites, and viruses. This test does not yield a pathogen. Since the symptoms do not improve, Thomas presents in our specialized outpatient clinic. We see a slim, yet well-trained patient in a slightly reduced general condition. We take a detailed history and order a blood exam. In addition, we schedule an upper and lower endoscopy. The upper endoscopy shows mild gastritis. This is a finding that is frequently observed, even in asymptomatic patients. However, the duodenum shows mucosal abnormalities, especially prominent vascularity and an irregular surface structure. Biopsies are taken from the duodenum and stomach. The colonoscopy is normal and reveals no signs of inflammation. Meanwhile, the results of the blood tests are available. The bloodwork shows mild anemia, a subnormal value for folic acid and the trace element zinc. The antibodies to the celiac disease autoantigen tissue transglutaminase are highly increased, eightfold above the upper normal value. The histological examination of the biopsies, taken during upper endoscopy, confirms the diagnosis of celiac disease, by showing a subtotal to total villus atrophy and crypt hyperplasia (stage Marsh IIIb to IIIc) and an increased number of intraepithelial lymphocytes (60, normal <25/100 intestinal epithelial cells). With the clearly established diagnosis of celiac disease, we inform the patient immediately about the necessity of a strict gluten-free diet. In addition, our dietitian gives him detailed instructions how to maintain the strict gluten-free diet and provides him with information about the gluten-content of common foods and the availability of gluten-free products. She also connects him to the national celiac society that is organized in local support groups and that is a forum for exchange between patients as well as between patients and experts. The celiac societies organize educational events and give regular updates on novel research on the disease. Thomas is prescribed folic acid and zinc-salt for 4 weeks to substitute his deficiencies. Initially, he has some difficulty to completely avoid bakery products and pasta. But after a few weeks, he gets along quite well with gluten-free products, including bread and pasta made of gluten-free cereals. In particular, he realizes that only after a few days of the gluten-free diet, his diarrhea started to disappear, and his overall wellbeing that was also impaired by fatigue and abdominal pain has improved. To his surprise, he realizes that with the gluten-free diet, he feels even more energetic than he felt before the acute enteritis. We see him again 3 months after the diagnosis. He reports continuous wellbeing and has regained 10 lb of body weight. He also tells us that his wife and two daughters had joined him in the gluten-free diet. His bloodwork now shows a disappearance of his anemia, a normalization of this folic acid and zinc levels, in line with his physical improvement. He is scheduled for the next follow up in 1 year.

Comment on Thomas H.
Thomas H. (48 years) is a typical and relatively common celiac patient: an adult who suffers from an acute intestinal infection that does not resolve after a few days up to a maximum of 2–3 weeks, as is common for most viral or bacterial infections. In this vein, the analysis of his stool samples 2 months after the onset of his diarrheal illness does not show common pathogenic viruses or bacteria. Obviously, an acute viral or

bacterial enteritis had triggered a severe form of celiac disease with weight loss, anemia, and nutrient deficiencies. It is very likely that he had low-level celiac disease before that did not markedly affect his health or wellbeing. Apart from improving on the gluten-free diet, he realizes only in retrospect that he feels better and more energetic than before the enteric infection. This is a common experience in patients with newly diagnosed celiac disease and no overt symptoms, who are often detected by family screening. Right at diagnosis, we had also recommended that Thomas' family be tested for celiac disease using the blood test for antibodies to tissue transglutaminase, since up to 15% of first degree relatives of celiacs also have the disease. This test turned out to be negative for his wife and his two daughters of age 8 and 13. Still, the daughters have an increased risk to develop the disease later in life.

4.2.2   Patient Martha-Ann (2 Years): Failure to Thrive

Martha-Ann (2 years) is Julia and Christopher M.'s first child. During her first year, Martha-Ann developed normally and was an agreeable and happy infant. At the age of 15 months, however, the situation gradually changed. Martha-Ann became increasingly cranky, could no longer sleep through, screamed at night, and was difficult to comfort. She had abdominal bloating, combined with phases of diarrhea and constipation. Feeding became more and more difficult, and Martha Ann's height and weight no longer developed according to her age. The pediatrician determined the celiac antibodies. The titer of the antibodies to tissue transglutaminase was increased tenfold. The doctor assumes that the diagnosis was celiac disease, but wanted to have an endoscopy performed by a pediatric gastroenterologist for a final proof. When the doctor informed the parents about the procedure, they were reluctant, because the endoscopic procedure had to be performed under anesthesia and Martha-Ann's condition was worrisome. The pediatrician understood the parents' concerns well, looked for alternatives, and got in touch with us. We can inform her that, according to the recent international guidelines of the Society of Pediatric Gastroenterology and Nutrition (ESPGHAN), a confirmation by endoscopy and biopsy is not needed when the serum autoantibody levels to tissue transglutaminase are elevated at least tenfold. The parents are relieved that the procedure can be omitted. The girl is immediately set on the gluten-free diet and her symptoms improve dramatically within only 1 week. After 3 months, Martha-Ann has gained weight, reaching almost her normal weight for age. Her belly-pain, bloating, stool irregularities, and crankiness have completely disappeared. We recommend that her parents also be tested for celiac antibodies. It turns out that Julia has a twofold increased antibody to tissue transglutaminase, whereas Christopher's test is negative. With an only mildly increased antibody test, the likelihood that Julia has celiac disease, too, is high, but confirmation is needed. Therefore, an upper endoscopy is performed. In contrast to small children, for adults, an upper endoscopy is not a stressful procedure. Usually, adults only need mild sedation, and the procedure is completed within 5–10 min. The endoscopy confirms moderately active celiac disease with partial villus atrophy (Marsh IIIa). The entire family goes on a gluten-free diet. Julia, who has never experienced any symptoms, notices that on the gluten-free diet, she is less fatigued and more energetic. Despite her diagnosis of mild celiac disease, her routine labs indicated no abnormality.

Comment on Martha-Ann

Martha-Ann (2 years) has a classic course of celiac disease in infancy. Infants usually develop classical symptoms, such as failure to thrive often combined with abdominal bloating and pain, stool irregularities, weight loss, sleeping and feeding problems, and crankiness. Usually, the symptoms develop with formula diets containing gluten or discontinuation of breastfeeding and introduction of solid foods. In this case, the diagnosis is established quickly, even without endoscopy. According to the new international diagnostic and treatment guidelines, celiac disease is considered to be confirmed when the celiac autoantibodies are elevated at least tenfold, and the infant's symptoms improve on the gluten-free diet. Therefore, in Martha-Ann's case, confirmation by endoscopy is not needed. This is a typical case of pediatric celiac disease. It is also often seen that one of the parents, most frequently the mother, transfers the major genetic predisposition for celiac disease (HLA-DQ2 or HLA-DQ8) to her child and is affected herself, as is Julia, Martha-Ann's mother. In contrast to her daughter, her disease is mild and appears asymptomatic. Nonetheless, the mother's wellbeing has improved on the gluten-free diet.

4.2.3   Patient Stephany G. (34 Years): Infertility

Stefany G. has just turned 34. She works as a project manager for an international pharmaceutical company where she coordinates clinical studies. She and her husband, Daniel, have been married for 5 years and have a strong desire to start a family. However, so far, all attempts to get pregnant remained unsuccessful. They presented in a fertility center where they were thoroughly examined. All results turned out to be normal. Hormone therapy was ineffective. In a training seminar, Stephany's gynecologist had learned that celiac disease could be a cause of infertility and gets into touch with us for further information. We see a healthy-appearing patient with normal body weight and no history of abdominal pain or discomfort and who reports overall physical and psychological wellbeing. The physical examination is normal. Nonetheless, we order the blood test for celiac disease, i.e., antibodies to tissue transglutaminase. To the couple's surprise, the test comes back positive. The diagnosis is confirmed by an upper endoscopy that shows mild macroscopic abnormalities. The biopsies from the duodenum reveal partial villous atrophy (Marsh IIIa), confirming the diagnosis of celiac disease. Stephany receives a thorough dietary consultation and immediately begins with the strict gluten-free diet that she finds inconvenient in the beginning, the more so since she does not feel any change in her wellbeing. Moreover, she and her husband also very much enjoyed eating sandwiches and Italian pasta. Nevertheless, both are motivated to continue with the gluten-free diet and are slowly getting used to the dietary change. After half a year, the titer of the celiac antibodies has dropped to normal. Stephany's long-standing mild anemia that was attributed to her strong menstrual bleeds had normalized. Eight months after having started the gluten-free diet, Stephany becomes pregnant. The pregnancy is uneventful, and the patient gives birth to a healthy girl in the 41st week.

Comment on Stephany G.

Stephany G. (34 years) presents with superficially asymptomatic celiac disease. She has no complaints, performs well, and is in no way physically compromised. She only has mild anemia, a common finding among women of childbearing age, especially when they have severe menstrual bleedings. This is not necessarily indicative of celiac disease. In the case of Stephany, however, the anemia has improved with the gluten-free diet. This can be explained by a form of malabsorption that mainly affects the uptake of iron, an essential component of hemoglobin in the red blood cells, in patients with otherwise asymptomatic celiac disease.

The course of the patient is particularly pleasing for the couple, as their desire to start a family has been fulfilled thanks to the gluten-free diet. It has long been known from large clinical studies that untreated celiac disease can lead to infertility, especially when it is accompanied by malabsorption. The underlying mechanism has not been fully explored. It is hypothesized that autoimmune reactions in the uterus and placenta that can occur in untreated celiac disease are the reason. Another hypothesis suggests that the coeliac autoantibodies to tissue transglutaminase prevent the implantation of the egg or the growth of the embryo. With the gluten-free diet, these antibodies decrease within a few months, and the couple is blessed with a successful pregnancy.

4.2.4   Patient Gregory M. (62 Years): Refractory Celiac Disease

Gregory M. is 62 years old and teaches English, history, and sports at a public high school. He is a popular and engaged teacher. Nevertheless, he is looking forward to his retirement in 3 years. Since his own children had left home several years ago, he and his wife are engaged in community work that they would like to extend after his retirement. For the past 6 months, however, Gregory had increasingly developed watery diarrhea, with up to eight bowel movements a day. His wife was deeply worried since her already very slim husband had lost 11 lb in the last 3 months. Moreover, he realized a drop in his performance but had been trying to ignore it. Finally, he saw his primary care physician who did not find any gross abnormalities on physical exam but arranged for some lab tests. The patient did not report any fevers or chills. The tests revealed mild anemia, and his stool samples were negative for pathogenic bacteria or viruses. The PCP referred him to a gastroenterologist for further medical work-up. An upper endoscopy and a colonoscopy were performed. The normal colonoscopy ruled out a chronic inflammatory bowel disease (Crohn's disease or ulcerative colitis). However, the upper endoscopy showed macroscopic changes in the duodenum, suspicious of celiac disease. Histology examination of the duodenal biopsies showed a severe coeliac disease with complete villous atrophy (Marsh 3c). The autoantibodies to tissue transglutaminase were slightly elevated (twofold). Therefore, the diagnosis of celiac disease seemed to be straightforward. Gregory and his wife received an in-depth consultation on the gluten-free diet that they began immediately. Indeed, diarrhea improved but did not disappear completely. He continued to have 2–3 watery bowel movements per day. His weight remained constant but did not increase, and his physical performance remained at a low level. After another 6 months, his gastroenterologist performed an upper control endoscopy. The result of this procedure showed no macroscopic and microscopic improvement, i.e., inflammation and complete villous atrophy persisted. The initially slightly elevated antibodies had normalized. This time, further studies were performed. The biopsy samples were stained for specific immune cell markers and analyzed by a molecular genetic technique, the so-called T cell receptor PCR (polymerase chain reaction). This confirmed the suspicion of refractory celiac disease, i.e., a form of celiac disease that is unresponsive to the gluten-free diet. The gastroenterologist then turns to us for advice on how to best treat this rare condition. We recommend prescribing the corticosteroid Budenoside as well as a commonly used immunosuppressive drug, Immuran, that contains the agent Azathioprine. This treatment is highly effective. Within a few days, Gregory's bowel movements normalize, and after two more months, he has regained his original body weight. His performance has also improved, and he feels as good as before his illness began. Another control endoscopy is performed showing that the inflammation of the small intestine has also improved significantly, but significant villous atrophy (now Marsch 3b) persists. Unfortunately, 9 months later, the original symptoms of weight loss, diarrhea, and drop in performance have returned. Special tests are performed again, and show similar results as before the pharmacological treatment was started. His gastroenterologist contacts us again and we recommend the prescription of a stronger immunosuppressant drug, Cladribine, which is used in the treatment of leukemias. This treatment change leads to a new improvement that is maintained for another year up to now. Cladribine, that is taken as a pill, has no pronounced side effects in most patients. Gregory and his wife can resume their active lifestyle and look forward to a happy retirement.

Comment on Gregory M.

Gregory M. (62 years) shows a characteristic course that is compatible with a newly manifested celiac disease at an advanced age. Such cases are not unusual in the gastroenterological practice. However, the patient only responds incompletely to the gluten-free diet, and after a few months, his general condition and symptoms worsen again, although he continues to adhere to the strict gluten-free diet. His specialist does just the right thing: he performs another endoscopy with extensive tissue sampling for advanced testing, including molecular genetic studies and special stainings. These tests confirm the suspicion that the patient, in fact, has refractory celiac disease, i.e., a therapy-resistant form of celiac disease that does not respond to the gluten-free diet. In Gregory's case, refractory celiac disease type 2 is diagnosed. In this form, the T cells have begun to multiply in the absence of nutritional gluten. The process has similarities to a T cell lymphoma, a severe immune cell cancer. Fortunately, Gregory has not developed such a lymphoma, but a condition that may develop into it. Based on the performed tests, an intestinal T cell lymphoma, the so-called EATL (enteropathy-associated T cell lymphoma), cannot be completely ruled out. Therefore, we arrange for a computerized tomography of the abdomen, that luckily does not show greatly enlarged lymph nodes in the abdominal cavity. An intestinal T cell lymphoma would have been accompanied by such enlarged abdominal lymph nodes. Taken together, the diagnosis of a refractory celiac disease type 2 could be established.

Based on this diagnosis, the patient is started on a relatively mild therapy, Budenoside and Imuran, a treatment that is usually well tolerated. Unfortunately, the improvement with this therapy only lasts for 6 months. Therefore, Gregory is given a stronger drug, Cladribine, that controls the disease up to the present day. Nonetheless, Gregory is at risk to develop the dreaded intestinal T cell lymphoma on top of his refractory celiac disease type 2. Refractory coeliac disease type 2 is mainly diagnosed in patients 40 years and older. A French study demonstrated that approximately 50% of patients develop EATL within 5 years. Although there are no proven treatments for this form of lymphoma, case reports show successful treatment in a minority of patients.

Background Information: Treatment of a Malignant Complication of Celiac Disease

Chris Mulder from Amsterdam, NL, reported cases of successful treatment of EATL by autologous stem cell transplantation. This is a therapy in which the patient's own blood stem cells are harvested. Subsequently, the patient receives very strong chemotherapy, which eradicates the patient's own hematopoietic (blood-forming) system, primarily in the bone marrow and the intestinal tissues—and thus the source of the lymphoma. The previously harvested blood stem cells are then returned to the patient by an infusion and start to repopulate the hematopoietic organs as well as the intestine, to develop a rejuvenated hematopoietic system, this time without the malignant immune cells. This therapy is usually applied to patients with advanced lymphomas and leukemias. In addition, another therapeutic approach is currently being tested in the US and Europe. Patients receive infusions with antibodies against the cytokine interleukin-15. Interleukin-15 is a central growth factor for the malignant lymphocytes whose growth is inhibited by the antibody. In the field of lymphoma treatment, we are facing rapid scientific and clinical development. Therefore, any prolonged remission of the disease can bring patients closer to a cure. Gregory M. suffers from a severe disease that until 15 years ago would have run a dismal course. With novel therapies that include the chemotherapeutic drug Cladribine, the situation has improved. However, these therapies are, at best, a bridge to better, potentially curative treatment. Refractory celiac disease or its advanced stage EATL are extremely rare overall and affect less than 1% of celiac patients diagnosed in adulthood. Importantly, the longer the gluten-free diet is maintained, the more the risk of developing refractory celiac disease type 2 or EATL approaches that of the normal population. This finding underlines, why maintaining the gluten-free diet is also important for celiac patients who have no or mild symptoms.

Background Information: Refractory Celiac Disease Type 1
Refractory celiac disease type 1 is about 10 times more common than the complicated type 2. Type 1 patients often have classic symptoms like abdominal pain and diarrhea and show elevated autoantibodies despite the gluten-free diet. In contrast to refractory celiac disease type 2 or EATL, the intestinal immune cells are not malignant. Experts hypothesize that patients with refractory celiac disease type 1 are particularly sensitive towards tiny amounts of gluten that often cannot be excluded, even on a strict gluten-free diet. Patients can usually be treated with low doses of Budenoside, the corticosteroid that is primarily active in the intestine.

4.2.5 Patient Paula K. (22 Years): Celiac Disease Combined with an Autoimmune Disease

Paula K. (22 years) is a dedicated biology undergraduate. Type 1 diabetes was diagnosed when she was 4 years old. Her diabetes had been well controlled with regular insulin injections. Meanwhile, she used a subcutaneous insulin pump that spared her the injections. She always coped well with her disease. Since she exercised regularly, her insulin requirements were low. More recently, however, the daily insulin dosing had become increasingly complicated. Her blood glucose levels fluctuated greatly, giving her the feeling that they needed to be controlled continuously, which had compromised her wellbeing and quality of life.

She visited her diabetologist, who could not find a cause for the worsened blood sugar control. Paula had noticed general discomfort and mild nausea that she attributed to the stress caused by her difficult-to-adjust diabetes. Fortunately, the diabetologist had attended a training-course for continuous medical education where he learned that patients with celiac disease and type 1 diabetes often have brittle diabetes, i.e., a difficult-to-adjust blood sugar. He, therefore, contacts our outpatient clinic. We advise him to determine Paula's tissue transglutaminase antibodies. They indeed turned out threefold elevated.

An upper endoscopy is performed for final confirmation: Paula has active coeliac disease, histological stage Marsh 3b. She is surprised that another disease had caused blood sugar fluctuations. We recommend that she follows the strict gluten-free diet. For Paula as a diabetic, this is easier said than done. The diabetes diet she has been following for many years is already restrictive, especially when she is eating out or meeting with friends. An additional gluten-free diet makes everyday life even more complicated. However, the gluten-free products that are now available almost everywhere make this task easier than 20 years ago. Our dietician supports her to adjust to the novel diet. Since Paula has been conscious about diet from early on, she quickly adjusts and copes well with her novel, more complicated nutritional needs. After only a few days without gluten, her diabetes becomes controllable, and the blood sugar fluctuations have disappeared. Paula can slowly return to an (almost) normal daily life and concentrate on her studies as before.

Comment on Paula K.

Paula K. (22 years) has insulin-dependent type 1 diabetes, an autoimmune disease of the pancreas, an organ that produces the blood sugar-regulating hormone insulin. Autoimmune disease means that the body's own immune cells, primarily the T cells, target the body's own organs and fight them like an invader. In the case of type 1 diabetes, T cells target the islet cells of the pancreas that produce insulin. The result is the destruction of islet cells and thus the loss of insulin production. As a result, the body's cells are no longer able to absorb glucose, the sugar that is the major fuel for the cells. The glucose that cannot be taken up by the cells due to the lack of insulin remains in the bloodstream. Only a minor part of the excess glucose is excreted via the urine. When patients are not treated with insulin, the excessively elevated blood sugar levels lead to severe complications including vascular disease like atherosclerosis, retinopathy, renal failure, and diabetic coma. In the long run, if the blood sugar is not optimally adjusted with insulin and regularly controlled up to four times a day, usually done by the patient, the risk of chronic disease is highly increased.

Numerous clinical studies show that, depending on the country and region, between 3 and 12% of celiac patients have at the same time type 1 diabetes. Conversely, a similar percentage of patients with type 1 diabetes have—an often unrecognized—celiac disease. As a type 1 diabetic, Paula is at a 1:20-risk of being affected. The question remains: why has it developed just now? Celiac disease in type 1 diabetes may remain undetected for a long time, as it can run a very mild course. Ill-defined environmental influences (like antibiotics and other medications or enteritis) can lead to a sudden deterioration that can either manifest itself with abdominal symptoms or the worsening of other preexisting diseases. In the case of Paula, such worsening manifested with the development of brittle diabetes. She had a mild intestinal inflammation due to celiac disease in the absence of abdominal symptoms. Her celiac disease was the reason for a reduced and irregular uptake of nutrients through the small intestine. The resultant fluctuations of the blood glucose levels were not easily controlled with her usual doses of insulin. With the healing of the intestinal inflammation and the improvement of nutrient uptake, a better blood glucose control with insulin was achieved.

Background Information: Paula's Autoimmune Family

In addition to the gluten-free diet we recommend that her parents and both of her younger sisters be tested for celiac disease autoantibodies. The rationale is that up to 15% of first-degree relatives of celiacs have celiac disease themselves. Often their celiac disease is mild or superficially asymptomatic. The family has now become alerted, and all family members visit our outpatient clinic for celiac disease and autoimmunity. Both parents have no celiac auto-antibodies—a finding that largely rules out celiac disease since they are consuming a gluten-containing diet. The mother has the diagnoses of autoimmune thyroid disease, Hashimoto's thyroiditis, that is treated with thyroid hormone substitution. Hashimoto's thyroiditis is an autoimmune disease in which the body's own T cells target the thyroid gland, causing an inflammation that is usually not painful, but that destroys the hormone-producing thyroid cells. The result is a low level of thyroid hormones. The clinical symptoms are, among others, fatigue, a lack of drive, and dry skin. These symptoms can be misdiagnosed as a mild depression. Other symptoms can be edema and severe constipation.

As mentioned, both parents had negative celiac autoantibodies on a normal, gluten-containing diet. With this finding, active celiac disease can be ruled out in at least 95% of subjects. However, if a person with celiac disease lives gluten-free for a long time, the celiac antibodies are usually no longer detectable in the blood. The half-life—the time that elapses before a value has dropped by 50%—is 1–2 months for celiac autoantibodies. This means that a patient who has a tenfold increased value at the time of diagnosis needs at least 6 months on the gluten-free diet until the value reaches the normal range.

Paula's sisters, who also consume the gluten-containing diet equally have normal celiac autoantibodies. We determine their thyroid hormone levels. The youngest sister shows a slightly decreased level of the thyroid hormone thyroxin (T4) and an increased level of the hormone TSH (thyroid-stimulating hormone), a constellation that indicates hypothyroidism (compromised thyroid function). Hashimoto's thyroiditis is confirmed by elevated thyroid autoantibody levels. We prescribe a daily pill of thyroid hormone and a small amount of a selenium salt for 3 months. Selenium substitution has been shown to be beneficial in the early stages of Hashimoto's thyroiditis. With this therapy, her performance in school improves and her lack of drive disappears that was interpreted as a symptom of puberty by the parents. Paula's family is a typical case of a family in which only one member has celiac disease, but other autoimmune diseases are present. Studies show that first-degree family members of an index patient with celiac disease have a high risk to develop celiac disease themselves as well as other autoimmune diseases, both with a probability of 10–15%.

Thyroid diseases and type 1 diabetes are common celiac-disease-associated autoimmune diseases. This is due to the fact that the genetic predisposition for celiac disease—HLA-DQ2 or HLA-DQ8—is also a prerequisite for these autoimmune diseases. Up to 30% of adult celiac patients have one or more, often undiagnosed, autoimmune diseases. Once a case of celiac disease is diagnosed, other family members should be tested. Families with celiac children should be aware that it is possible to assess the risk to develop type 1 diabetes. There are four specific diabetes autoantibodies that can be determined in the blood. If none of these antibodies is detected, there is no risk. If 2 antibodies are detectable, the risk is high, and the doctor will recommend the family to have the blood sugar levels checked on a regular basis since early treatment can beneficially affect the course of the disease. Type 1 diabetes is manifest, once 3 of these antibodies are positive.

Background Information: Autoimmune Families in General

In celiac families, the risk of autoimmune diseases is greatly increased. Relevant autoimmune diseases are:

- Autoimmune thyroid diseases with decreased secretion of thyroid hormone (Hashimoto's thyroiditis) or excessive secretion of thyroid hormone (Grave's disease)
- Type 1 diabetes as found in Paula's case
- Psoriasis and other skin diseases, especially the blistering dermatitis herpetiformis
- Rheumatoid diseases, such as rheumatoid arthritis, scleroderma, and psoriasis arthritis
- Autoimmune hepatitis and others (see also Table 4.2)

From the clinical point of view, every celiac patient and all first-degree relatives should be examined for autoimmune diseases. Conversely, if a patient suffers from one of these autoimmune diseases, the patient should be tested for celiac disease by determination of transglutaminase autoantibodies.

4.2.6 Summary of the Celiac Cases

We describe five characteristic cases that shed light on the broad spectrum of celiac disease and its associated comorbidities. The cases illustrate the diversity and complexity of this disease, often surprising even for experts. For this reason, it is not surprising that there are still many misdiagnosed or undiscovered cases. The need for information for those affected is still enormously high. However, it should be noted that the majority of diagnosed cases of celiac disease are benign and that most patients get along well with the gluten-free diet. They do not have an increased risk of serious complications. Patients with celiac disease receive valuable support for their daily living via their celiac societies. A list of the major celiac societies is available via the following links: For Europe: https://www.aoecs.org/members, for the US and outside of Europe: https://www.aoecs.org/international-coeliac-organisations.

Chapter 5
ATI Sensitivity

5.1 Wheat Sensitivity: What is it Exactly?

While some people still question the existence of any form of wheat sensitivity that is not celiac disease, there is no scientific doubt that there are even various forms of non-celiac wheat sensitivity (NCWS). A substantial number of patients is familiar with the symptoms as their complaints are tightly linked to the consumption of wheat products. Understandably, these patients feel slandered when NCWS is derided in public, also among health care professionals, and depicted as a mere fad. From a medical point of view, NCWS is a diagnosis of exclusion, since celiac disease and classical wheat allergy have to be ruled out. Based on the most recent scientific evidence, we can now clearly define that NCWS includes two inflammatory conditions. These are the newly discovered ATI-sensitivity and the atypical wheat allergy. With 10–15% and 4%, respectively, both of them are highly prevalent and important.

5.1.1 Differential Diagnoses of the Wheat Sensitivities

The most relevant differential diagnosis that needs to be ruled out is celiac disease. It is largely excluded by a negative blood test for autoantibodies to tissue transglutaminase. Usually, an endoscopy with tissue sampling from the upper small intestine is required for confirmation. When these findings are negative, the question remains if the patient's complaints are related to a (classical) wheat allergy. The tests for classical wheat allergy are discussed in Chap. 7. Patients with such an allergy show the clinical picture of immediate reactions, i.e., within minutes up to 1 h after consumption of the allergen, in this case, wheat. Those reactions can be sneezing, asthma, redness, irritation or itching of the skin or mucous membranes. Also, gastrointestinal complaints, such as abdominal pain

© Springer Nature Switzerland AG 2019
D. Schuppan, K. Gisbert-Schuppan, *Wheat Syndromes*
https://doi.org/10.1007/978-3-030-19023-1_5

and diarrhea, can occur. Symptoms become apparent immediately after wheat consumption and cease quickly once wheat is discontinued. Classical wheat allergy is an inflammatory reaction and often a serious condition. Its prevalence is well below 1% of the total population, and therefore, it can be considered a relatively rare allergy.

Apart from classical wheat allergy, we have recently identified an atypical allergy to wheat and other common foods. These atypical allergies that are more frequent than classical food allergies are extensively described in Chap. 7. Notably, the most important allergen of atypical food allergies is wheat, in 60% of the cases, followed by milk, soy, and yeast. An atypical wheat allergy (usually) becomes symptomatic with a delay of a few hours with abdominal pain, diarrhea or constipation as predominant symptoms. Most of these patients have received the diagnoses of irritable bowel syndrome (IBS). IBS is a diagnosis of exclusion when no other causes for the abdominal complaints are found. Up to now, reactions to food have not been considered relevant causative factors of IBS. Treatment recommendations are generally very much focused on factors like stress reduction and regular meals that are often of little help. We now know that atypical food allergies cause the symptoms in more than 70% of IBS patients. A clear-cut diagnosis of these food allergies is presently only possible by means of a special endoscopic procedure, but dietary exclusion and re-exposure are also valid and helpful diagnostic tools (see Chap. 7).

Apart from the atypical wheat allergy, the quantitatively most prominent and most important category of NCWS is ATI-sensitivity. Again, an immediate reaction—as many might think– is not a characteristic feature of ATI-sensitivity. In our pre-clinical and clinical studies, we have shown that the majority of affected patients have complaints and symptoms outside the gastrointestinal tract and basically show a worsening of pre-existing chronic conditions. Our clinical experience with a large number of patients on two continents also confirms that it is precisely patients with serious chronic diseases who accordingly benefit from an ATI-free, i.e., a wheat-free diet. These comprise diseases as diverse as chronic inflammatory bowel diseases, multiple sclerosis or rheumatic disorders, including connective tissue diseases like scleroderma. In addition, ATI aggravate fibrotic diseases that develop with chronic inflammation, prominent examples for which we could show this effect of ATI are liver fibrosis, scleroderma, and lung fibrosis.

5.2 ATI Stimulate the Innate Immune System

When we in our research group searched for inflammatory proteins in wheat that could be the cause of NCWS, we exclusively found non-gluten proteins, namely amylase-trypsin-inhibitors (ATI). ATI are a family of at least 11 related proteins that comprise approximately 3% of the wheat proteins (see Sect. 2.3). This is much less than the gluten-proteins that amount to 80–90% of the proteins in wheat. Yet, when ingested, this little quantity is sufficient to activate cells of the intestinal innate immune system. This induces an only mild intestinal inflammation. The crucial point is that this mild inflammatory stimulus has no or minimal consequences in healthy subjects, but potentiates pre-existent inflammation in patients with modest to severe chronic conditions. These far-reaching findings were very unexpected and differ dramatically from prior research on the course of NCWS. Despite these novel discoveries, even today, many researchers and clinicians find it hard to deviate from their original research path and clinical conceptions. Therefore, we briefly describe prior research and the paradigm change that our novel findings are bringing about in the following paragraph.

Prior studies that had investigated intestinal tissue samples of patients with NCWS indicated mild signs of immune activation by using refined technology. At that time, scientists had also observed that extracts containing wheat proteins or impure gluten could elicit an innate immune response in cultivated intestinal biopsies of patients. Based on these weak results, they concluded that gluten is the culprit in NCWS. However, many of these results were not reproduced by scientists from other research groups. Moreover, a central requirement in immunology was not met, i.e., a target receptor for gluten was not identified. Therefore, the cause and mechanism of the immune activation remained unclear, and many researchers doubted that such innate immune stimulation existed at all. In our laboratory in Boston, funded by the National Institutes of Health (NIH), we set out to unambiguously identify both, the stimulus and the receptor. Initially, for 2 years, we screened the myriads of gluten proteins to find one or more candidates that would show activity to stimulate innate immunity. To our disappointment, we were unable to detect such activity among the gluten proteins. We then turned to other protein components of wheat and, after painstaking research, discovered a completely different class of wheat proteins with such immune stimulatory activity: the class of amylase trypsin inhibitors (ATI). The family of ATI exclusively stimulate the key innate immune cells, namely monocytes, macrophages, and dendritic cells. They bind to the toll-like receptor-4 (TLR4), according to the key-lock principle. TLR4 is predominantly located on these innate immune cells and is probably the most important and central receptor of the innate immune system. TLR4 became notorious as a mediator of the toxic shock syndrome when bacterially contaminated tampons caused sepsis in women. Normally, the TLR4 on the immune cells serves as a sensor for dangerous bacteria, recognizing an important bacterial cell wall component: lipopolysaccharide (LPS). It is the more surprising that these wheat proteins, the ATI, that we ingest with our daily nutrition also activate TLR4. However, this activation is significantly weaker and therefore, only leads to a mild inflammatory reaction in the intestine that cannot be detected with conventional endoscopy or conventional histological studies. On closer inspection, inflammatory cells of the intestinal wall are slightly increased after contact with ATI. These inflammatory cells are not counted in routine diagnostics. After contact with ATI, the innate inflammatory cells up-regulate so-called activation markers on their surface. These markers are also not assessed in standard diagnostics. Activation markers are proteins that are present on the surface of inflammatory cells, once they have been stimulated. They can be visualized in tissue samples using specific antibodies. ATI from wheat and related gluten-contain-

- a family of 11 related non-gluten proteins in wheat
- small compact proteins, each with 124-168 amino acids
- form monomers, dimers and tetramers
- major ATI: CM3, CM17, 0.19, 0.28, 0.53
- play a role in wheat grain germination
- represent ca. 3% of wheat protein, 0.3% of wheat flour dry weight

- compact structure, not inactivated by digestive proteases
- activate the receptor for bacterial lipopolysaccharide (LPS) = toll-like receptor 4 (TLR4) on intestinal immune cells
- thereby inducing a low grade intestinal inflammation

- prominent immune stimulatory activity only by ATI in gluten containing cereals
- ATI content in wheat is dependent on variety and cultivation
- commercial gluten (vital gluten etc.) contains up to bis 5% ATI

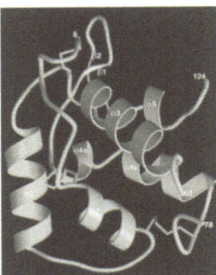

X-ray structure of ATI 0.19 with 4 α-helice (spirals) and 5 intramolecular disulfide bonds (Oda Y et al, Biochemistry 1997)

Fig. 5.1 Characteristics and functions of wheat ATI. The unique molecular structure endows the wheat ATI with a high resistance to degradation by intestinal proteases. This allows them to effectively activate the intestinal innate immune cells via toll-like receptor 4

ing cereals are thus the only known nutritional molecules that can activate this central immune receptor, TLR4. The following figure summarizes the central features of the ATI-induced immune activation (Fig. 5.1).

5.3   ATI: An Unexpected Cause with Great Effect

How is it possible that an agent that causes an only mild inflammation in the gut, an inflammation that is not even visible by standard endoscopy, leads to a diversity of severe symptoms in the periphery? Our recent scientific studies have demonstrated how this works. If we give a single dose of purified ATI to mice[1] that had been on an ATI-free diet before, we can see an immediate activation of innate immune cells in the entire intestine, i.e., from the upper small intestine to the rectum within 2–12 h. This ATI-effect is replicated when mice are fed the same amount of ATI within standard wheat flour, that contains many different proteins, including gluten, and carbohydrates. In contrast, a 30-fold higher amount of purified gluten, without ATI, does not have any pro-inflammatory effect. Taken together, these studies clearly demonstrate that it is the ATI, and not gluten or other wheat components, that activate the innate immune system in the living organism. Notably, it is well established that between mice and man, there is no significant difference in the TLR4 signaling

---

[1] The mice won't get hurt when they receive ATI in their diet. All experiments have been evaluated and approved by the Animal Care Committees in Boston or the state of Rhineland-Palatinate and considered to be fully ethically justifiable and necessary for the improvement of human health.

in general and in the ATI response in particular. Therefore, we are in a unique and lucky situation where mouse experiments and data can be transferred to human health and disease with no restriction.

5.3.1   Cells of the Innate Immune System Leave the Gut to Promote T Cell Activation

To our surprise, the ATI-induced immune activation was several-fold higher in the lymph nodes surrounding the intestine than in the intestine itself, as we have shown in our studies. It is important to know that the lymph nodes play a key role as meeting points of innate immunity and adaptive immunity, i.e., the T cells. Since ATI feeding only leads to mild inflammatory signs in the gut, but to significant activation in the surrounding lymph nodes, we can conclude that the innate immune cells must quickly leave the gut towards the lymph nodes after their activation by ATI. In the lymph nodes, they have an effect on the T cells that regularly pass through them via the bloodstream. According to our hypothesis about the mechanism of how ATI worsen chronic disease everywhere in the body, some of the circulating T cells that pass through the lymph nodes originate from the organs affected by chronic inflammation. These are T cells that maintain the chronic inflammation, originating, for example, from the joints in rheumatoid arthritis or from the central nervous system in multiple sclerosis. This mechanism would also come into play in chronic inflammatory bowel diseases (IBD), i.e., diseases of the intestine itself. In IBD, as in all inflammatory conditions, the T cells would return to their organs of origin after their passage through the lymph nodes. The contact with the ATI-activated immune cells from the intestine makes these T cells more aggressive than they had already been. This explains why wheat and specifically ATI worsen chronic inflammatory diseases. It also explains why we cannot measure inflammatory activity in the intestine itself with conventional methods: because the key immunological processes take place in the lymph nodes, outside of the gut, where the innate immune cells migrate after their ATI-induced activation in the gut. Figure 5.2 shows these complex relationships.

5.4   The Gut as Key Regulator of Immune Balance

Apart from their clinical impact, these findings highlight a general principle of high importance. The intestine and the intestinal immune system do not only modulate intestinal but also extra-intestinal health and inflammatory diseases. ATI-sensitivity superbly illustrates this paradigm, i.e., a defined nutrient elicits a signal in intestinal inflammatory cells; this signal is transported to the surrounding lymph nodes, where they encounter inflammatory T cells from the periphery. These T cells home back to their organ of origin to exacerbate the inflammation.

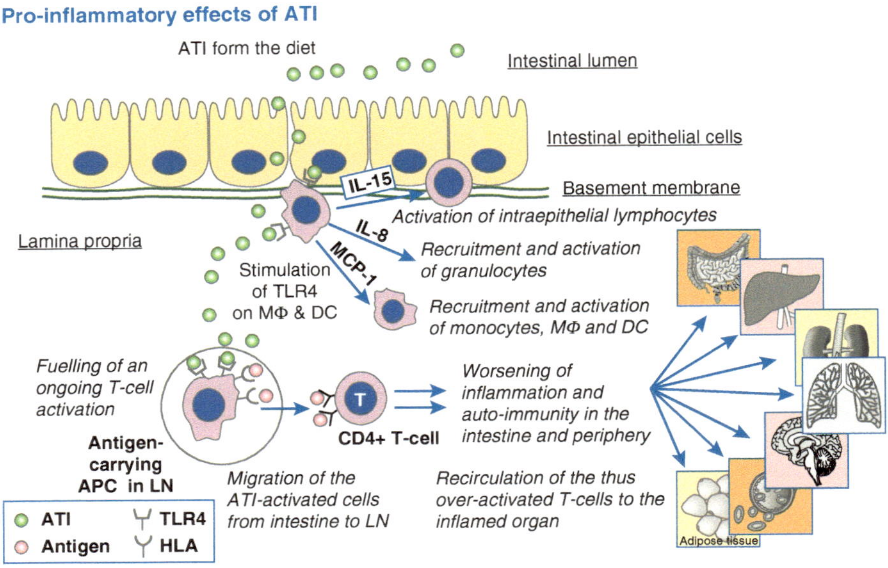

Pro-inflammatory effects of ATI

Fig. 5.2 Inflammatory effect of ATI. ATI remain largely undigested and therefore biologically active in the gastrointestinal tract. Their uptake is both via active and passive resorption through the intestinal epithelial cell layer, after which they reach the underlying connective tissue (lamina propria), where they activate cells of the innate immune system, mainly dendritic cells (DC) and macrophages (MΦ), by binding to toll-like receptor 4 (TLR4) on their surface. Thus activated, these cells secrete inflammatory cytokines and chemokines such as interleukin-8 und -15 (IL-8, IL-15), or macrophage chemotactic protein-1 (MCP-1) that further recruit and activate innate immune cells, especially monocytes from the blood that then mature to tissue resident MΦ and DC. Our data indicate that these immune cells, once activated by ATI, can leave the gut towards the surrounding lymph nodes (LN) where they generally promote antigen presentation via antigen presenting cells (APC, mainly DC) and therefore T cell activation. This explains our findings that nutritional ATI enhance ongoing chronic diseases inside and outside of the gut, including adipose tissue inflammation, autoimmune and metabolic diseases

Apart from the elucidation of this pathway, there is a tremendous complexity in the interaction of the gut with the periphery. Thus, the gut as the largest immunological organ of the body is continuously confronted with numerous substances from food as well as countless bacteria and their metabolic products. Research on the effect of gut bacteria and their metabolites on the body's immune system in health and disease has recently gained momentum, with many unsolved questions.

In this context, our research data show that ATI do not only activate innate immune cells but also directly change the intestinal microbiome towards a state of dysbiosis, i.e., pro-inflammatory and disease-promoting bacterial populations in the gut. These two additive mechanisms explain the strong effect of ATI on chronic inflammatory diseases. In a larger context, the surprising and far-reaching effect of ATI may not stand alone, and other yet to be identified nutrients may have disease-promoting, but also disease-preventing effects. In our opinion, ATI are the cornerstone that brought the topic of general nutrition from grandma's kitchen wisdom into the limelight of serious science and medicine. In contrast to common nutritional advice, we are dealing with defined, biologically active molecules. To identify those components in nutrients is an important topic of our current research. However, the ATI stand out, since a large part of the world's population consumes huge amounts of wheat—100–400 g of wheat flour per day—and other foods containing gluten and thus ATI. ATI lead to a slight immune activity in everybody, including healthy people, and thus to an inflammatory response in the gut. In healthy people, this seems to be relatively unproblematic, but patients with chronic diseases, i.e., 10–15% of most populations, suffer from a worsening of the already active inflammatory processes in the body due to ATI.

5.5 "Gluten-Free" is Largely "ATI-Free"

ATI are found in all gluten-containing cereals, i.e., not only in wheat, but also in barley, rye and the ancient forms of wheat: spelt, emmer and einkorn. Our ongoing research has shown that most of all gluten-free foods are nearly ATI-free (Fig. 5.3). That means that for all ATI-sensitive patients, there is a dietary rule of thumb: Avoid gluten-containing cereals and cereal products! In this sense, it is important to know that patients with ATI-sensitivity do not have to adhere to the gluten-free diet as

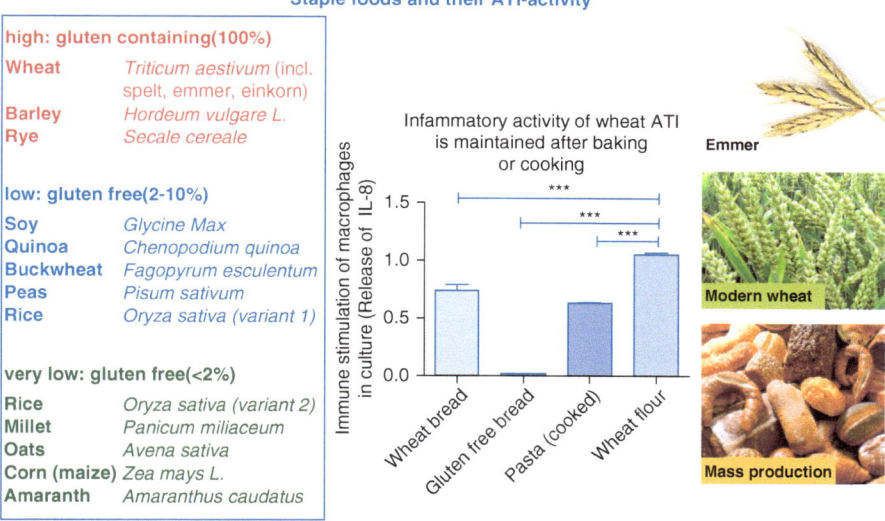

Fig. 5.3 Plant derived staple foods and their ATI activity. The immune stimulatory ATI activity can be determined by their quantitative liquid extraction from staples and foods, followed by a test that is based on activation of macrophages in cell culture. These extracted ATI dose-dependently activate the macrophage toll-like receptor 4 (TLR4), and lead to secretion of inflammatory mediators such as the measured interleukin-8 (IL-8). Gluten containing grains and goods, here a standard wheat flour, has been set as 100% (full activity), although ATI content and activity can vary significantly depending on (wheat) variety and site of cultivation. Notably, ATI activity is only slightly reduced by baking or cooking. Gluten free products are usually very low in ATI activity

strictly as required for patients with celiac disease and for patients with (typical and atypical) wheat allergy. The reason is that the damaging effect of ATI is dose-dependent. Based on the current state of research and our clinical experience with patients, a 95% reduction in daily ATI consumption should be sufficient and safe to prevent adverse effects. A 95% ATI-reduced diet can be achieved by avoiding all obvious sources of gluten as well as undeclared refined foods and ready-made meals. This diet is much easier to follow compared to the 100% gluten-free diet that Patients with celiac disease and wheat allergy have to adhere to.

Remember
The damaging effect of ATI is dose-dependent. For ATI-sensitive patients, we recommend a 95% reduction of gluten-(=ATI-)containing foods.

5.6   Most of "Gluten Sensitivity" is ATI-Sensitivity

Based on the findings described above, the term "gluten sensitivity" cannot be further upheld. The gluten and ATI-contents of foods are merely associated but not identical. Gluten and ATI are two very different classes of molecules. Importantly, while the gluten content of wheat variants remained constant over hundreds of years, the ATI-content is highly variable. Our preliminary results in projects with wheat breeders and cereal scientists indicate that ancient wheat variants contain lower quantities than modern wheat, but also show that the ATI-content among different modern wheats can differ at least by a factor of 3. Basically, all plants and cereals have molecules that resemble wheat ATI, but these molecules do usually not activate the TLR4 receptor in the gastrointestinal tract. As we have found in our studies, related proteins from other plants with similar functions for the germination and growth process do not show this activity.

The fact that the ATI have such an effect in gluten-containing cereals must probably be regarded as a mere coincidence. We reject the popular statement that ATI or enhanced amounts of gluten or even novel ATI or gluten genes have been intentionally bred into modern wheats or even introduced by genetic manipulation to increase yield or pest resistance. These incorrect statements are often propagated in the media.

The association of gluten and ATI is the reason why many clinicians and researchers with interest in wheat sensitivities wanted to stick to the concept and diagnosis of "gluten sensitivity", although they are beginning to realize that gluten is not the cause of NCWS. In this context, the alternative term "wheat sensitivity" can also be misleading, because is too unspecific. As we have learned, there are now three quite different and well-defined forms of sensitivity to wheat as well as related (gluten-containing) cereals. These are

1. celiac disease
2. typical and atypical wheat allergy
3. ATI-sensitivity.

All these diseases have in common that they are inflammatory. To differentiate these three entities is crucial, in order to reach a clear diagnosis and initiate an appropriate dietary therapy. One reason for some clinical and research colleagues to stick with the old term "gluten sensitivity" was that the term "wheat sensitivity" would exclude the other gluten and ATI-containing cereals, mainly rye and barley. Nonetheless, we use the term "wheat sensitivities" *pars pro toto* for all gluten- and ATI-containing cereals for two reasons: Firstly, wheat in European mythology is the mother of all grains, guarded by the goddesses Demeter and Ceres. In ancient Greek and Roman artworks they are often depicted with ears of wheat or barley. This illustrates that early on, wheat (and barley) were assigned a dominant role in human nutrition. Secondly, the wording "wheat sensitivity" distinguishes wheat and related cereals from the essentially gluten- and ATI-free, mostly non-European cereals, like corn, rice, oats, quinoa, and amaranth.

Note

⇨ What has been propagated as "gluten sensitivity" in bestselling books and the media does not exist. Instead, a clear diagnosis of ATI-sensitivity or the two forms of wheat-allergy has to be made. Our research undoubtedly indicates that the era of undifferentiated and misleading buzzwords in the context of wheat is over now.

5.7   ATI: A New Paradigm in Immunology

The discovery of ATI as immune stimulators has generated several scientific, immunological, and clinical innovations that are unique and have never been described before. These novel insights will thoroughly change the future research and clinical landscape, comparable to the change that the discovery of tissue transglutaminase as autoantigen of celiac disease brought to the field of immunology. In the following, we want to illustrate these changes and their significance in detail.

5.7.1   Discovery of Tissue Transglutaminase as Autoantigen of Celiac Disease

Our research report on the identification of tissue transglutaminase as autoantigen of celiac disease that we published in Nature Medicine in 1997 is the most cited paper in the field until today and is regarded as a paradigm shift among experts. With this discovery:

1. it was shown for the first time that an autoantigen modifies the external trigger—gluten—in such a way that it can elicit a strong immune reaction in the body
2. a blood test could be developed to reproducibly diagnose celiac disease as a disorder which is the most common chronic inflammatory intestinal disease

3. celiac disease was defined as an exemplary disorder of the immune system in which an external trigger has to interact with a genetic predisposition and the identified autoantigen to cause disease.

Background Information: Autoantigen

An autoantigen (antigen = antibody generator) is a body's own protein (sometimes also a carbohydrate or lipid) that induces an endogenous immune reaction, usually via antibody production. Normally, the immune system is educated to ignore the body's own proteins. The tolerance towards the body's own molecules and therefore cells and tissues is broken in autoimmune diseases. Different characteristic autoantigens play a role in various autoimmune diseases. Their essential importance lies in the fact that they trigger an immune reaction in the body that leads to the production of autoantibodies that are characteristic of a given autoimmune disease and detectable in the blood. These autoantibodies are important diagnostic tools to confirm a certain autoimmune disease, but usually have no pathogenic activity themselves. Examples of autoimmune diseases that can be diagnosed by their autoantibodies in the blood are diseases of the thyroid gland, the liver and the joints (rheumatoid arthritis). The actual organ damage in autoimmune diseases is caused by the destruction of own cells and tissue by organ- and cell-specific T cells, usually CD4+ T cells.

5.7.2   Discovery of ATI as Immune Stimulators: Another Paradigm Shift

Another paradigm shift is the discovery of ATI as general immune stimulators. This discovery has triggered a new way of thinking that especially affects the fields of immunology and nutritional sciences. The following points are decisive for this paradigm shift:

1. ATI are the first known food proteins that activate *innate* immunity in the intestine. Until now, only proteins were known that activate *adaptive* immunity, i.e., T cell immunity, in the intestine. No other protein has comparable effects on existing or developing diseases.
2. A receptor for ATI has been identified that mediates this immune reaction. This is the TLR4 receptor on innate immune cells. TLR4 is probably the most important and central receptor of the innate immune system. This aspect is extremely important. Science requires so-called specificity, i.e., proof of the underlying mechanism. In case of ATI-sensitivity, the mechanism is based on the identification of the receptor that transmits the signal to the cell. Something comparable has never been shown for any other food molecule.[2]

---

[2] All authors that incriminated gluten as trigger of innate immunity did neither identify defined gluten peptides nor a specific receptor. The lack of these specific identifications is a grave problem

3. ATI are proteins that are mainly left untouched by the gastrointestinal enzymes. There are only a few other known biologically active proteins with a similar enzyme resistance. ATI reach all parts of the intestine, from the upper small intestine to the rectum, and remain active throughout, exerting their disease-causing effects over the whole length of the gut.

4. Another novelty is that the primary activation of the TLR4 receptor by ATI in the intestine does not only stimulate the innate immune cells but that these innate immune cells, in turn, activate the adaptive immune system (T cells) that had already been activated in other ongoing diseases. Thus, ATI do not only trigger an immediate reaction but also enhance the T cell reactions in pre-existent diseases. This means that two regulatory loops interact: The loop of the innate immune system via the TLR4 receptor and the loop of T cell immunity within the setting of an already existing chronic disease. The T cell reaction is aggravated by the activated innate immune cells that in turn had been activated by ATI. Such an interaction between two regulatory loops induced by a nutritional component has never been shown before.

5. Contrary to the public view, but also prevailing expert opinion, ATI do not primarily cause gastrointestinal symptoms, but lead to a worsening of existing diseases, especially outside of the digestive tract. Considering traditional thinking, it may be difficult to grasp that the site of contact is different from the site of end-organ damage. Even when the gastrointestinal tract is affected, as in chronic inflammatory bowel disease, the promotion of the intestinal inflammation by ATI is secondary: The T cells become activated in the surrounding lymph nodes and then migrate back to the gut.

6. For the first time, we identified a clearly defined pathway that points to dietary intervention that can improve a large number of chronic diseases. These are chronic diseases that could previously only be controlled with expensive and potentially side-effect-prone drugs.

Note

⇨ With the discovery of ATI, we have identified a component of the normal daily diet that seriously interferes with the human immune system and worsens chronic diseases. The unusual and unexpected feature of this mechanism is that neither patients nor clinicians realize the connection of ATI-consumption with their illness, since ATI-effects are not immediate and wheat consumption is common and taken for granted. When patients eliminate ATI-containing foods from their diet they usually recognize the connection, because their condition improves.

---

and not acceptable in serious scientific research. Having not identified the players in the game renders any kind of statements on cause and effect invalid or speculative.

5.7.3   ATI Promote Obesity and Associated Diseases

Another surprise of our research was the finding that ATI promote obesity and fatty liver disease. As in autoimmune diseases, this effect is more pronounced in people who already suffer from metabolic syndrome. In terms of obesity, our animal experiments suggest that the ATI-effect can amount to a difference of 10% bodyweight on the longer term. This means that a person weighing 100 kg (220 lb) could easily reach a body weight of 90 kg (198 lb) on the ATI-reduced diet without a change of total calories consumed. This obesogenic effect of ATI (that do not have a caloric value on their own) is dose-dependent, i.e., mild with low dose and severe with a high dose of ATI. For some time, we could not explain this effect despite an otherwise equal consumption of food calories. Only recently we discovered that, apart from the inflammatory activity, ATI also directly change the microbes of the gut. The result is a so-called *dysbiosis*, i.e., an increase in potentially harmful bacteria at the expense of beneficial bacteria. In particular, the ATI-induced bacteria increase the digestion of otherwise non-digestible carbohydrates and therefore increase the so-called energy harvest. This increase in nutrient extraction from the food can explain the observed weight gain.

A number of well-performed studies have shown that a 10% weight loss in overweight people usually leads to a highly significant improvement in their metabolic state. This includes a significant reduction of the risk to develop type 2 diabetes or even a normalization of the diabetic state; a reduced risk for cardiovascular diseases, including myocardial infarction and stroke, and for fatty liver inflammation (nonalcoholic steatohepatitis, NASH) that may result in liver cirrhosis and liver cancer. This improved metabolic state through weight loss can also be confirmed in the blood, especially via reduced levels of fasting glucose and lipids, and of inflammation markers. The increased inflammation in obese people has its origin in the adipose tissue and the liver, but also in the blood vessels. The negative metabolic effect of ATI is particularly enhanced by a modern lifestyle with a hyper-caloric diet and reduced physical activity.

5.7.4   Modern Eating Habits and the Obesity Epidemic

In view of the obesity epidemic, ATI are gaining importance. The prevalence of obesity (body mass index, BMI > 30) has dramatically increased in most developed and developing countries. For example, today more than 30% of the US population is obese, compared to about 10% 40 years ago (Fig. 5.4). In most European countries, as well as in China, India, the United Arab Emirates, and almost all other former developing countries, that have seen a rapid economic and social change in the last two to three decades, the number of obese people has doubled to tripled. While one of the reasons is an oversupply of food combined with a decrease in physical activity, another cause are changes in eating habits towards highly refined

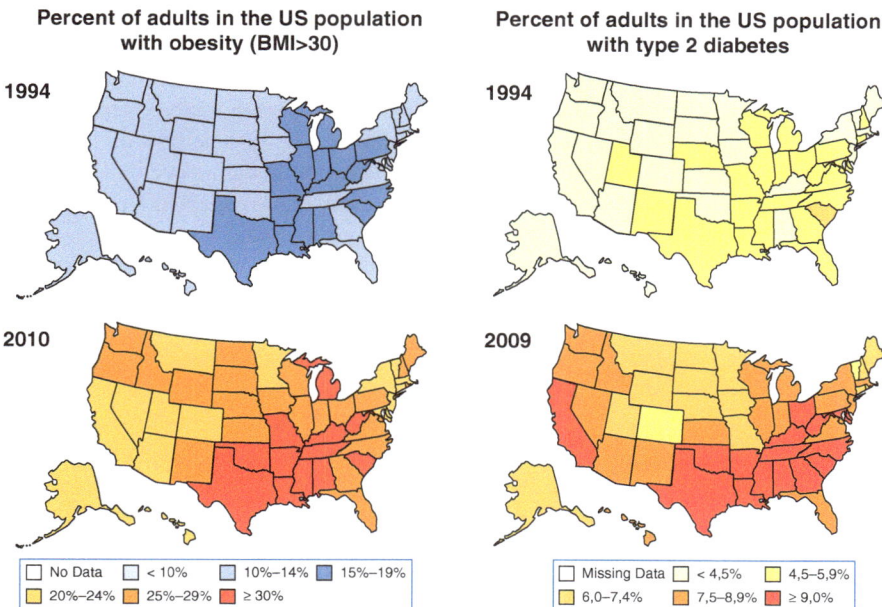

Fig. 5.4   Dramatic increase in obesity and type 2 diabetes. These data show that the prevalences of obesity and type 2 diabetes have dramatically increased in the US, and that their increase goes in parallel. Similar trends are found in most parts of the developed and developing world. Illustrations are from the Centers of Disease Control, www.cdc.gov

and artificially composed foods. These include products enriched with high fructose corn syrup (fructose-glucose-syrup), whose use in food manufacturing has increased 50-fold in the last 30 years and that is now found in almost all industrially produced foodstuffs. Here, the excessive use of fructose as a sweetener is significantly responsible for the increase in obesity, since fructose is directly converted into body fat if it is not quickly burnt by physical activity. Also, fructose is not perceived as satiating to the same extent as traditional sugar (sucrose and glucose) and is therefore easily consumed in excessive amounts. Cells take up fructose by a specific surface transporter protein (glut5) that does not require the hormone insulin. This is the reason why fructose was previously used as sugar for diabetics but was removed from the shelves since it was recognized that for type 2 diabetics, who are overweight anyhow, fructose further enhanced obesity.

5.7.5   Complex Foods

Since fructose is a major sugar in fruit, one may ask why it should not be harmful there to the same extent. The answer is that raw, unprocessed fruit, like all natural foods, can be regarded as a complex matrix. Complex foods have a positive effect on metabolism. Intestinal absorption of refined foods is accelerated (simple matrix). One prominent unfavorable effect of these foods is that the carbohydrates are already partly cleaved due to the processing and therefore readily available, leading to a rapid increase of the blood glucose. In contrast, a complex food matrix ensures a gradual uptake and metabolism of the nutrients. This is associated with numerous advantages. Thus, the resorption of the nutrients by the intestine occurs slowly and step by step, since most of them must first be cleaved or liberated from the food matrix by intestinal enzymes. This is particularly important when it comes to the major source of energy, namely sugars and starch. They are metabolized differently, depending on how quickly they are available as fuel. An excessive build-up of blood sugar due to rapid resorption of sugar and starch from refined foods is largely converted into body fat. In contrast, a low-level increase of blood sugar for a prolonged time, as occurs with the consumption of complex foods, will largely be used as fuel for the cells and not stored as body fat. In addition to the beneficial effect on sugar uptake, complex foods also contain micro-nutrients that counterbalance pro-inflammatory signals from the gut, such as elicited by ATI. For example, certain fruits, vegetables, and spices contain anti-inflammatory molecules that antagonize the pro-inflammatory TLR4 receptor. This has been shown for cinnamon, but we also found such activity in other food components, e.g., in hops. Finally, complex foods contain a multitude of trace elements, vitamins, and vitamin-like substances, such as antioxidants, that are vital for the body's functioning and have beneficial effects on metabolism. In refined foodstuffs, most of these components are missing with unfavorable consequences.

Background Information: Rapid Increase of Blood Glucose
Normally, the regulation of blood glucose works as follows: The small intestine resorbs the glucose supplied by the food. It is then transferred to the bloodstream where the elevated blood glucose signals to the islet cells of the pancreas to release the hormone insulin. The released insulin reaches the body cells via the bloodstream and transmits the signal to take up the glucose. The cells then use the glucose as fuel for their functioning. If supplied in excess the cells transform the glucose into the storage carbohydrate glycogen, mainly in the liver. When the glycogen stores are full (at around 400 kcal, equivalent to 90 g glucose), the blood sugar is converted to fat that is stored as fat droplets in the liver cells (hepatocytes), but also in the fat cells (adipocytes) of adipose tissue.

5.7.6   Glucose and Insulin

In the case of glucose, this leads to a rapid release of insulin from the pancreas. The released insulin enters the bloodstream and ensures that glucose is quickly absorbed by the body cells. But as rapidly as the insulin level has increased, it also drops. This rapid drop in insulin creates a sense of hunger a short time after the meal with refined carbohydrates and leads to new craving, although the glucose of the prior meal has not been burned. Instead, the glucose has been incorporated as body fat. The extent of insulin release after ingestion of a defined amount of food calories is called *glycemic index*. The glycemic index is particularly high after ingestion of refined foods. The insidious nature of these foods not only leads to overeating and increased fat storage, but in the long term also promotes a serious condition called insulin resistance. Once insulin resistance has developed, the body cells no longer react adequately to the insulin stimulus and no longer efficiently absorb glucose from food. Glucose that now floods the blood without being removed by insulin-sensitive cells continuously overstimulates the pancreatic beta-cells to release even more insulin—in a futile attempt to make the cells responsive again, in order to burn or store the excess blood glucose. Thereby, the normally well-functioning regulatory circle of glucose uptake and removal is aborted. If this derangement persists, patients develop type 2 diabetes.

Patients with type 2 diabetes have consistently elevated blood glucose levels, despite permanently increased insulin levels. The patients' cells, namely cells that normally absorb glucose, especially liver and muscle cells, lose their ability to react adequately to blood insulin. The ever-increasing insulin levels are the only way for the body to bring glucose from the blood into the cells where it is used as fuel or stored as fat. Despite these derailments, type 2 diabetics do often inject additional insulin to overcome the resistance. The consequence is more weight gain, further promoting the vicious circle. This is in stark contrast to patients with type 1 diabetes who have a severe insulin deficiency and who need additional insulin to survive. The insulin sensitivity of patients with type 2 diabetes can only be increased again by 2 measures. First, patients need to increase their physical activity that enhances the insulin sensitivity of the muscle cells as well as the liver cells. Boosting muscle mass and muscle activity is a highly efficient measure to increase insulin sensitivity. Second, patients should lose adipose tissue mass, whose amount correlates with insulin resistance.

As a rule of thumb, the higher the amount of adipose tissue, the greater is the insulin resistance. Insulin resistance is further aggravated by the inflammatory properties of adipose tissue. Here visceral (internal abdominal) adipose tissue has the strongest pro-inflammatory potential. The combination of both measures—more exercise and loss of fat mass—is highly efficient, since it best increases the ratio between muscle mass and adipose tissue, thereby allowing the body cells to regain their insulin sensitivity. Type 2 diabetes, formerly known as diabetes of the elderly, no longer occurs only in older patients, but frequently in younger people and even children. In addition, the metabolic derangement of type 2 diabetes is not only limited to elevations of blood sugar and to obesity but also has severe consequences far beyond. These patients usually also have

- dyslipidemia, that is high blood lipid and cholesterol levels, increasing the propensity for atherosclerosis, vascular thrombosis, stroke, hypertension, and myocardial infarction,

– a fatty liver up to fatty liver inflammation (NASH) that can lead to liver cirrhosis and liver cancer, and
– an increased general cancer risk.

The metabolic derangement described above, highlights the problem that nowadays in view of the many denatured and refined foods we cannot and must no longer rely on our feeling of hunger and satiation. Statements in the media and in talk shows that propagate that the body naturally knows what it needs are misleading and wrong. The equally often voiced suggestion that some overweight is not harmful or even healthier than being slim is also utterly wrong, unfounded, and dangerous. This idea may have contained a grain of truth in history when natural foods were consumed, and physical work was the rule. In our times, however, it is grossly misleading, since the body composition, such as the muscle to fat ratio, and therefore the metabolic signals have changed in the vast majority of contemporary people. The newly discovered form of body fat, the so-called adipose tissue organ, consists of inflammatory adipose tissue and is due to refined foods, overnutrition, and a lack of physical activity and exercise.

5.7.7   Inflammatory Body Fat: The Adipose Tissue Organ

In the last 2–3 decades, the average ratio of fat to muscle mass has shifted significantly towards fat. This has led to fewer muscle cells that burn off carbohydrates and fat. This has been accompanied by a marked increase not only of the peripheral, subcutaneous but especially by the visceral, the "bad", internal belly fat. This visceral adipose tissue exerts a negative influence on metabolism and develops its own dynamics, justifying to speak of an adipose tissue organ. One of the peculiarities of the adipose tissue organ is that it contains excess inflammatory cells. Due to the inflammatory cells, this adipose tissue organ is in a permanent state of low-grade inflammation that the subject does not sense. The inflammatory cells release cytokines and other messenger molecules into the blood that act on the whole body, including the blood vessels and the liver. They promote vascular pathology, such as arteriosclerosis, myocardial infarction, and stroke, as well as liver inflammation. The liver itself stores fat and develops into a fatty liver with inflammation, increasing the risk of cirrhosis and liver cancer. The technical term for this relatively new but already very common liver disease is non-alcoholic steatohepatitis (NASH). In the US and the UK, the number of people affected by fatty liver is about 30% and those with the severe form, NASH, about 4%. In most other countries of the world fatty liver ranges between 10 and 30% and NASH between 2 and 4%.

Figures 5.5 and 5.6 illustrate the mechanism of adipose tissue inflammation due to over-nutrition and the detrimental consequences for the entire body.

Adipose tissue inflammation (1)

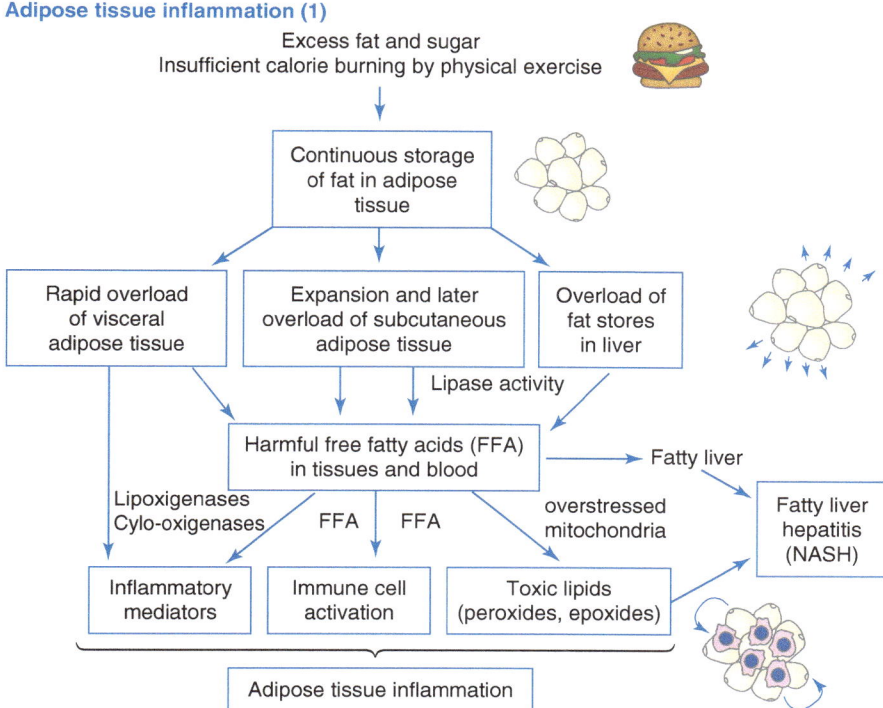

Fig. 5.5 **Mechanisms of adipose tissue inflammation** (**1**). An increased consumption mainly of refined carbohydrates (sugar) overburdens the capacity of adipose tissues and the liver for their uptake, transformation to and storage as lipids. An increased activity of lipid cleaving (lipolytic) enzymes (lipases) leads to enhanced cellular, tissue and blood levels of free fatty acids (FFA, fatty acids that are nor esterified with glycerol). These FFA induce (innate) inflammatory responses, damage the major metabolic liver cells (hepatocytes) and increase the cells' insulin resistance and therefore reduce the uptake of glucose from the bloodstream, leading to type 2 diabetes. Moreover, they promote inflammation of adipose tissues and the liver, resulting in nonalcoholic steatohepatitis (NASH)

5.7.8 Role of ATI in Obesity and Metabolic Syndrome

In view of the above dynamics, we hypothesized that the high ATI content in today's hyper-caloric and refined nutrition should have an additive effect on inflammatory processes in adipose tissue and related pathologies. It would therefore not be surprising if an ATI-containing diet would contribute to fatty tissue inflammation. We could indeed prove this assumption in mouse experiments. Mice were fed small amounts of ATI together with a typical modern diet containing refined carbohydrates with a high glycemic index and high-fat content over 8 weeks. The ATI

Adipose tissue inflammation (2)

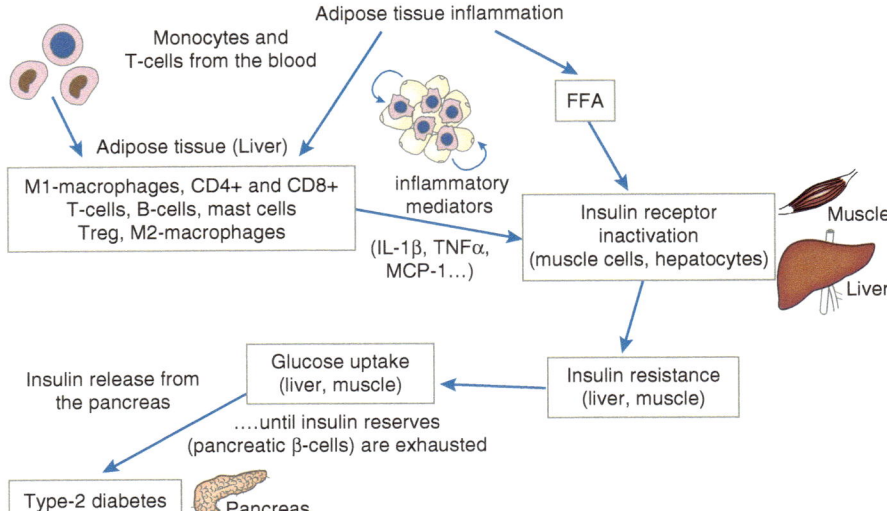

Fig. 5.6 Mechanisms of adipose tissue inflammation (2). The inflammatory reaction of the adipose tissue and the liver is caused by a local activation of immune cells that attract further inflammatory cells from the bloodstream via release of chemoattractant chemokines and cytokines. This creates a milieu where the usually present anti-inflammatory M2-type macrophages and regulatory T cells (Treg) are suppressed. The increased circulating free fatty acids (FFA) and inflammatory mediators inhibit the effect of insulin on muscle cells and hepatocytes, major utilizers of glucose, via inflammatory inactivation of insulin receptor signaling. Thus, the insulin that is secreted from the pancreas, even if produced in excess, cannot keep pace with the excess of glucose that needs to be taken up by the cells. This creates a state of insulin resistance that is the basis of insulin-resistant (type 2) diabetes that is usually associated with obesity and a lack of physical exercise. The therapy of choice is sustained weight reduction and physical exercise that increases energy consumption and muscle mass, all factors that can normalize insulin sensitivity, improve cardiovascular health and stop liver inflammation and fibrosis

amounted to less than 0.15% of the total food, i.e., it was calorically irrelevant. Animals fed the identical diet, but without ATI, served as controls. The animals that received the ATI gained 10% more weight than the controls. Their visceral adipose tissue increased threefold, and the liver fat-content twofold. Both, the visceral adipose tissue and the liver, showed significantly more inflammation than in the ATI-free control mice, and they developed more pronounced insulin resistance and type 2 diabetes. We also investigated if gluten had a similar obesogenic and metabolic effect. To investigate this, the mice were fed a high surplus of pure gluten, 4% of the total food. The gluten fed mice did not gain weight or develop any metabolic pathology. These experiments clearly showed that minute amounts of ATI that are consumed with a normal, wheat-based diet, but not gluten, is responsible for the weight gain, type 2 diabetes, adipose tissue, and liver inflammation. To sum up, ATI generally increase the inflammatory state in the whole body and promote disease in any tissue that is already inflamed.

5.7.9   Consensus Meetings on Non-celiac Wheat Sensitivity

In recent years, more and more physicians have been confronted with patients complaining of wheat-related symptoms. The topic has increasingly been brought into the public so that a panel of interested scientists, clinicians, and dietitians convened in an attempt to untangle the many aspects of non-celiac wheat sensitivity (NCWS). The meetings were organized by Dr. Schär Company, the primary provider of certified gluten-free breads, pastries, bars, and flour in Europe. So far, 5 meetings of about 50 international participants, including our own group, have been organized in the years 2010, 2012, 2014, 2016 and 2018. Three meetings produced consensus statements that are available online (see commented references).

Accordingly,

1. NCWS is an inflammatory reaction of the intestine that is closely linked to the intake of wheat. The symptoms occur within a few hours up to 1 day after wheat consumption and disappear within a similar timeframe when wheat is discontinued. Based on prior studies that examined intestinal tissues of patients with NCWS, the panelists agreed on an underlying activation of innate immunity. Therefore, NCWS is not related to classical allergies or celiac disease that have to be excluded diagnostically.
2. Apart from intestinal symptoms, NCWS manifests itself with non-specific general symptoms, such as exhaustion, fatigue and lack of the ability to concentrate (foggy mind), as well as headache, skin eruptions, and joint- and muscle pain.
3. Using standard endoscopical and biopsy assessment, patients with NCWS do not show overt macroscopic or microscopic finding of intestinal inflammation.

With every novel meeting, this diverse panel slowly grasps the paradigm shifts of our scientific and clinical discoveries. Still, it is hard for many of the participants to dismiss two of their long-held favorite beliefs and convictions: (1) major complaints must be abdominal, (2) gluten must be responsible for NCWS.

These meetings can be seen as a typical example of how tedious it can be to implement real paradigm changes that are based on clear-cut empirical evidence, once a community with established preconceptions is involved. With the discovery of ATI-sensitivity, we have shown that the majority of patients with NCWS have complaints and symptoms outside the gastrointestinal tract. Our scientific findings in basic research and preclinical studies, as well as our clinical experience with a large number of patients on two continents, show that it is predominantly patients with serious chronic diseases who benefit from a wheat-free diet. These include diseases as diverse as chronic inflammatory bowel diseases, multiple sclerosis or rheumatic disorders, including connective tissue diseases like scleroderma. In addition, we have shown that most of the patients with irritable bowel syndrome (IBS) have an atypical wheat allergy whose symptoms completely disappear with the exclusion of wheat from the diet.

5.7.10   Are FODMAPs of Central Relevance? the Answer is No!

A new, broadly discussed topic that has recently led to new food products on the market is the so-called FODMAPs. We consider this hype as exaggerated and bluntly wrong. FODMAPs stands for fermentable oligo-, di-, monosaccharides and polyols. These are common carbohydrates in natural foods, especially vegetables, legumes, and fruits, but also grains. The FODMAPs in these foods are only partly resorbed by the intestine. The remainder is metabolized by the intestinal bacteria. This bacterial intestinal fermentation is a normal process that helps to maintain intestinal health. FODMAPs serve as food for beneficial bacteria and are the source of short-chain fatty acids that are important nutrients, especially for the intestinal epithelial cells. Therefore, FODMAPs are essential for the health of the intestinal microbiome and for the entire body.

There is no doubt that excessive consumption of FODMAP-rich foods can cause bloating, and occasionally belly pain or diarrhea. Think of eating half a watermelon, a pound of cherries, plenty of green beans or lentils, onions, cabbage and, to a lesser extent, wheat. Everybody is familiar with the resulting effects. In addition to the mentioned beneficial health effects, FODMAPs are anti-inflammatory. The anti-inflammatory effect is due to both, the FODMAP-dependent microbiome as well as the short-chain fatty acids.

It is well-established that some patients with an underlying intestinal inflammation and belly pain may feel relieved when they reduce FODMAPs in their diet, but this can be explained by the mechanical effect of reduced gas formation and bloating. This does not affect or treat the underlying disease.

There are some studies that demonstrate some symptom relief in patients with IBS. However, most patients with so-called IBS, in fact, suffer from an underlying and undiagnosed food allergy (see Chap. 7) and only identification and exclusion of the allergen lead to cure.

The recent hype suggests that a FODMAP-reduced or even FODMAP-free diet would be a magic cure for intestinal diseases. Unfortunately, many patients put their hope on this diet. We want to stress that the FODMAP diet

1. is unhealthy, since it is poor in fiber and it favors intestinal dysbiosis, a reduction of beneficial and growth of less favorable gut bacteria, as several studies have shown;
2. is disliked if not hated by patients, because it is highly unpleasant to abandon all the fresh and tasty foods that contain FODMAPs.

Most importantly, the FODMAP diet does not address the root of any serious inflammatory disease, but may rather worsen it. It is unethical if the FODMAP diet is implicitly propagated as a cure for severe diseases. Due to the commercialization campaign, many patients have developed misconceptions and believe that the FODMAP diet is a cure for their diverse abdominal complaints and their underlying disease. In our clinic, we see many distressed patients who have engaged in extreme FODMAP diets without substantial benefit. It is obligatory that foremost a serious underlying disease must be searched for. Since a modest reduction of FODMAPs is not harmful, everybody is free to experiment with the kind and amount of FODMAP-rich foods as long as the diet remains balanced where FODMAPs play an important role. In summary, the concept of FODMAPs is Potemkin villages. It pretends to the public that FODMAPs play a role in curing diseases when, in reality, there is not a single disease they can cure. At best, they ameliorate some intestinal symptoms.

5.8 Case Vignettes: Patients with ATI Sensitivity

5.8.1 Patient Carol S. (40 Years): Diffuse General Complaints

Carol S. is 40 years old and teaches at a public elementary school. She is married and has a son and a daughter of age 8 and 12 years. She tells us she always easily caught infections since early childhood. In the last 5 years, however, she suffered from frequent episodes of bronchitis and sinusitis, and she fears that this could be due to a severe underlying condition. She also complains of fatigue, muscle and joint pain, and poor concentration that she describes as foggy mind. She has seen many specialists who did not find any pathology. Her ENT doctor did not detect abnormalities of the sinuses, and her OB-GYN doctor ruled out premature meno-pause or other gynecological problems. She describes her marriage and her family life as balanced and harmonious and attributes any psychological distress to her compromised health. She also enjoys her work as a teacher, although it has recently been difficult for her to concentrate on teaching and to cope with the liveliness and exuberance of the children. To her own dismay, she has increasingly lost patience with the kids. In search for help, she surfed on the internet where she detected a "gluten-free" health blog. In the related chat, she received the recom-mendation to consult a natural healer, who advised her to start a strict gluten-free diet. To her great surprise, after a few days of the gluten-free diet, she felt much better. Especially the diffuse symptoms, like fatigue and foggy mind, but also the muscle and joint pain improved remarkably. Three weeks later, on vacation in Canada, she succumbed to the temptation of French baguette and fresh croissants. At the end of the vacation, Carol felt miserable. At home, she immediately resumed her gluten-free diet, and again, the symptoms of her illness improved within a week.

Carol S. now consults us, since she believes to have celiac disease. Her general practitioner is unconvinced since she does not complain about abdominal pain or diarrhea and does not show any lab abnormalities. He thinks that the improvement with the gluten-free diet is due to a placebo effect. We perform the tissue transglu-taminase antibody test that the GP did not order. The test turns out negative, indicat-ing that celiac disease is unlikely since Carol had consumed gluten-containing foods recently. Normally, in order to confirm the diagnosis, an upper endoscopy with tissue sampling from the duodenum is done. However, we first have an analysis of her genetic predisposition for celiac disease done, HLA-DQ2 and HLA-DQ8. This test is negative which unambiguously excludes celiac disease. We also test for a classical wheat allergy (the blood test for IgE-antibodies) that results negative, too. The negative allergy test, in combination with no symptoms typical for a food reaction, rules out a classical as well as an atypical wheat allergy (see Chap. 7). We diagnose ATI sensitivity by exclusion. This diagnosis is supported by the repeated improvement of her symptoms under the gluten/ATI-free diet and the worsening after the resumption of wheat ingestion. To ensure that Carol's general symptoms—such as joint and muscle pain—are not caused by another yet undiagnosed disease, we order additional antibody tests for autoimmune diseases like rheumatoid arthritis and systemic lupus. Fortunately, these are unremarkable. After our diagnosis of ATI-sensitivity Carol is relieved, since she felt already stigmatized as a "hypochondriac" or a "psycho-somatic case". With our diagnosis, she feels assured that she can justify her gluten/ATI-free diet in her family and in public. Moreover, she is relieved that she has to adhere only to the 95% ATI-reduced diet instead of pursuing the 100% gluten-free diet that is required in celiac disease. This less restricted diet makes adherence much easier, both in her family and when it comes to eating out since minor amounts of ATI are not harmful. The detrimental effect of ATI is dose-dependent, and we know from our studies that 5% of the normal daily consumption is not harmful.

Comment on Carol S.

Carol S. (40 years) suffers from non-specific symptoms that resemble permanent flu. She reports recurrent bronchitis and painful sinusitis as well as chronic fatigue, joint and muscle pain, and inability to concentrate. The symptoms significantly affect her quality of life but are not taken seriously by the many doctors that she visits, since her lab values show no abnormalities. After a natural healer advises her to try a gluten-free diet, Carol discovers a connection between her symptoms and ATI/gluten-containing foods. Initially, she cannot believe that her symptoms improve with this "fad diet" but learns that her problems quickly return after consumption of wheat. Her GP does not carry out the celiac disease antibody test since he reasoned that without belly pain and diarrhea celiac disease is unlikely. However, celiac disease frequently does not go along with abdominal symptoms, and patients mainly report so-called unspecific, i.e., extra-intestinal symptoms. We can exclude celiac disease with a negative antibody and genetic test, sparing endoscopy. Had the genetic test been positive, an upper endoscopy should have been performed, optimally after a renewed gluten challenge for at least 4 weeks. We can also exclude the second form of wheat sensitivity, wheat allergy since Carol has a negative blood IgE-test against wheat protein and does not report abdominal problems after wheat consumption. Therefore, the diagnosis of ATI sensitivity can be established. The renewed wheat exposure that led to a worsening of the symptoms, as well as the rapid improvement after resuming a wheat-free diet further support this diagnosis.

5.8.2   Patient Ester W. (36 Years): Crohn's Disease Since Adolescence

Ester W. (36 years) is a long-term outpatient at a center for chronic inflammatory bowel diseases (IBD). At age 16, she was diagnosed with ileal Crohn's disease; i.e., Crohn's disease located in the ileum, the terminal part of the small intestine where it joins the colon. Crohn's disease is a chronic inflammatory bowel disease with a genetic predisposition that leads to a strong inflammation of the colon, but also of the small intestine. In Ester's case, both the small intestine and a small part of the colon are affected. Since she was 16 years old, she repeatedly had to take a corticosteroid, a drug that suppresses the body's overactive immune system. She experiences her disease, the medication and its side-effects as extremely unpleasant, constraining, and stressful. During inflammatory episodes, she suffers from abdominal pain, diarrhea, bloody stools, and general symptoms with weight loss and a lack of wellbeing. In the past, disease-exacerbations required high doses of corticosteroids for many weeks that, in turn, induced severe side effects like edema and an elevation of her blood glucose. Therefore, her medication was changed to so-called biologicals. Biologicals are antibody preparations that reduce disease exacerbations and that worked well for Ester. Still, her life is profoundly influenced by the disease, and due to her impairments, she has not entered into a firm partnership or started her own family, as she would have loved to do. When we see her, she tells us that this is a considerable burden. She says that her job as a university librarian is acceptable, but not what she really wanted to achieve. She would have loved to major in literature and art history but felt unable due to her disease. Ester had tried many unconventional ways to cure her symptoms. Recently, she has read about dietary interventions on the internet. She presents in our clinic in order to discuss, if and how far her disease could be improved by dietary interventions, such as the so-called elementary diet.

First, we carry out some laboratory diagnostics that show normal values except for mild anemia. Ester had received her last medication (antibody infusion) 2 months ago, but she continues to lack drive and feels physically weak. Moreover, she has cramping abdominal pains lasting from 30 min to 1 h 2–3 times a week. Her last colonoscopy 6 months ago revealed a moderate activity of her inflammatory bowel disease. Having taken a brief dietary history, we find that the patient consumes a balanced diet, though with plenty of bread and other wheat-containing foods. Because ATI in the gluten-containing foods exacerbate inflammation, we recommend to abstain from gluten-containing foods and explain to her the ATI-reduced diet. After 6 weeks, we see the patient again. She reports that she feels significantly better and that her abdominal cramps have completely disappeared, despite no change in her medication. Still, she complains of a lack of wellbeing and a reduced general performance. We advise her to be patient and to stay with the ATI-reduced diet. We see her back 6 months later. This time she reports that she has never experienced such a long period of stable improvement. For the first time in many years, she feels full of energy and free of malaise. With the disappearance of the abdominal pain, and especially of her recurrent diarrhea, she could emotionally open up and entered into a love relationship for the first time in her life. She stresses how well it feels not to experience herself as being a burden for others and to be able to move freely without fearing sudden diarrhea or abdominal cramps.

Commentary on Ester W.

Ester W. (36 years) is a patient with Crohn's disease, an inflammatory bowel diseases (IBD). IBD, ulcerative colitis and Crohn's disease, are serious inflammatory diseases that to date can only be treated with drugs that suppress the immune system and thereby counteract the inflammation. The severe course of Ester's disease necessitates such medication. Her general wellbeing, her physical and psychological performance, and her quality of life are significantly affected by the disease itself as well as by the medication, up to the point that she had abandoned the idea of private happiness and having children. Her condition also blocked her educational and professional development. As many of these patients, she gathered information on alternative therapies and found several studies that report success with so-called elementary diets. Elementary diets are composed of low-molecular, hydrolyzed food components with very low allergenic or inflammatory potential. Such diets can effectively attenuate inflammation and symptoms in IBD. On the other hand, elementary diets are quite expensive, and their acceptance by patients is low since these formulas are often described as unpalatable "space food". We suggest a different approach, based on our findings that an ATI-reduced diet mitigates IBD. We give Ester our dietary advice about the ATI-reduced diet that is easy for her to follow – quite in contrast to the elementary diet.

The positive outcome with the ATI-reduced diet, even if full recovery can take several months, is compatible with our findings of the mechanisms how ATI amplify chronic inflammation, including IBD. Ester's is a typical case as we have seen many before. Still, on a larger scale, we are planning randomized controlled clinical studies to confirm the effect of the ATI-reduced diet in patients with IBD.

5.8.3   Patient Michael B. (54 Years): Multiple Sclerosis

Ten years ago, Michael B. (54 years) experienced visual problems that occurred all of a sudden and lasted for several hours. These episodes of blurred vision were accompanied by a feeling of general weakness. Such episodes were becoming increasingly frequent in the next months. His ophthalmologist did not find any abnormalities and referred him to a neurologist. After several studies, especially a magnetic resonance imaging (MRI) of the brain and a lumbar puncture, i.e., sampling of cerebral fluid from the lower spinal cord, the neurologist diagnosed multiple sclerosis (MS). Michael B., who works as a lawyer in his own law firm and who has a family with three school-age children, was hit hard by the diagnosis. At first, he perceived the diagnoses as a death sentence, especially professionally, and in his mind's eye, saw himself already sitting in a wheelchair in need of constant care. His neurologist explained to him that there are different forms of MS. Thus, the disease can run a slowly or non-progressive course, while a rapid progression that leads to invalidity in a few years is relatively rare. In addition, there are already a number of effective pharmacological therapies that slow down, and sometimes even stop the disease process in MS. Michael received such a drug, interferon-beta that is given subcutaneously three times weekly and appeared to work, but brought along flu-like side effects. Even if he did not feel well, at least the disease seemed to stabilize. Especially, the visual disturbances occurred less frequently, and Michael was able to continue his work as a lawyer. Unfortunately, after 8 months, he noticed an increasing general weakness. Everyday movements became difficult for him, such as climbing the two flights of stairs to his office. Moreover, he noticed insecurity in balancing his gait. His neurologist ordered a control MRI of the brain that showed enhanced white matter lesions, a sign of progression. At this point, the neurologist transferred Michael to our outpatient clinic for a consultation about supportive dietary options. He had heard about our pre-clinical and incipient clinical studies that demonstrate that an ATI-free diet has a beneficial effect on the symptoms of MS, while the consumption of ATI-containing foods worsens the course. Based on our studies, we recommend the patient to start the ATI-reduced diet. Michael and his wife receive a dietary consult, in which also the rationale of the ATI-reduced diet is explained to the couple. The whole family switches over to the ATI-reduced diet by replacing all cereal foods with gluten-free products. Although scheduled for a follow-up in our clinic after 2 months, the patient shows up after only 3 weeks to let us know how much his condition has improved. He tells us that he can again climb the steps to his office without having to pause and that he feels more energetic and confident overall. In another visit, after 6 months, he reports further improvement. Overall, he can follow his daily routine almost unhindered, with a mild remaining uncertainty of gait.

Comment on Michael B.

Michael B. (54 years) suffers from a serious autoimmune disease, multiple sclerosis (MS). In this disease, the T cells, i.e., the cells of the adaptive immune system, attack the body's own structures in the central nervous system (CNS). MS is an autoimmune disease of the CNS that leads to the destruction of the myelin sheath, i.e., the insulating layer of the nerve fibers. The myelin sheath is destroyed by the inflammation, disturbing or even interrupting the transmission of nerve impulses from the CNS, i.e., from the brain to the periphery and vice versa. One of the first manifestations of this process occurs in the optic nerve that runs almost completely within the brain from the occipital region to the eye. MS can progress very quickly and can lead to complete paralysis. More often, it develops gradually, and many patients show a relapsing-remitting course, thus experiencing deterioration, followed by some improvement. So far, our patient has had this milder form of MS. Unfortunately, there is still no easy way to predict the course of the disease. Michael's ocular symptoms are typically accompanied by general weakness and coordination disorders, especially gait insecurity. We recommend the ATI-reduced diet to the patient that he can easily implement with the support of his family. The recommendation is based on our studies that show a detrimental effect of ATI-containing diets on the course of this neurodegenerative disease. We have regularly observed improved neurological functions and enhanced physical and mental performance in patients with MS after they had embarked on the ATI-reduced diet. In order to further substantiate our observations, we have initiated a randomized clinical study in patients with relapsing-remitting MS. Here, disease activity, inflammation markers in the blood, physical and mental performance, and quality of life are major parameters for the efficacy of the diet. In Michael's case, as well as in other individual patients from our clinic, an improvement with the ATI-reduced diet was evident.

5.8.4 Patient Bruce K. (49 Years): Weight Gain and Incipient Type 2 Diabetes

Bruce K. is a 49-year-old carpenter who runs his own successful family business, established by his father, that he has expanded in the last 15 years. His business is going well but is demanding, with 60–70 working hours per week. Bruce is happily married for 22 years, and his three children are successful in their education and jobs. His primary care physician refers him to us, because of fatigue and elevated liver enzymes. The detailed medical workup[3] shows that he had gained 15 kg (33 lb) in the last 18 months. He tells us that he used to exercise and run regularly for an hour every morning over many years, but discontinued his exercise routine a year ago. He has not changed his eating habits, and no other family member experienced weight gain. He also feels exhausted quickly and less energetic and efficient than before. His family and employees have noticed that he became forgetful, often does not listen properly and seems to be distracted. His primary care physician diagnosed a mild depressive episode and prescribed an antidepressant that did not improve his condition. Bruce does not accept the diagnosis of depression and sees no trigger or other reason for being in this condition. Moreover, his PCP diagnoses an incipient type 2 diabetes (elevated fasting glucose), a lipid metabolic disorder (dyslipidemia, i.e., hypertriglyceridemia, hypercholesterolemia, high low-density, and low high-density lipoproteins) and recently also elevated liver enzymes.

Family history reveals that both grandmothers of the patient had type 2 diabetes at an older age. It is, therefore, likely that the family has a genetic predisposition for diabetes and other metabolic diseases that often are associated with type 2 diabetes. We find that his slightly elevated liver enzymes result from fatty liver,[4] which is confirmed by ultrasound. We have excluded other liver diseases through blood tests. Alcohol as the cause of the liver enzyme elevation and Bruce's fatty liver can be

---

[3] We reserve 30–60 min for each new patient, to take a detailed history, perform a thorough physical exam, and evaluate prior findings and medical records.

[4] In our outpatient clinic, we do not limit ourselves to intestinal or autoimmune diseases, but also consider all body systems that we further explore with special tests and studies, if indicated.

ruled out because the patient follows an abstinent lifestyle. His dietary history shows that he consumes a balanced diet, though with a relatively high amount of red meats and bread. With the finding of fatty liver, we do not proceed with a liver biopsy, as is often done, to rule out NASH or advanced liver fibrosis, but propose a dietary change first. Based on our research, we know that the intake of ATI promotes type 2 diabetes and fatty liver disease. Therefore, the patient and his wife receive dietary advice how to carry out the ATI-reduced diet. As a substitute for bread and other wheat-containing foods, the patient is advised to eat gluten-free products, which would not change his caloric balance, but improve his metabolic and adipose tissue inflammation. We also advise that to lose weight the overall consumption of (the gluten/ATI-free) starchy foods should be reduced by at least 50%. Bruce is relieved that we diagnose a likely ATI-sensitivity, and rule out a severe underlying somatic disease or depression.

We see the patient again after 3 months. His appearance has changed. He has lost 8 kg (17.8 lb) in weight and tells us that he has become more physically active and motivated, running three times a week again, which he did not feel able to do before. Moreover, he reports that his concentration and memory have improved significantly. He also realized a positive effect on his social environment and family. By omitting the bread that he normally consumed in excess, he has also cut down on other carbohydrates, which had an additional positive effect on his weight. Overall, adhering to the ATI-reduced diet has led to a remarkable improvement of his well-being. We see him again after another 6 months. This time he presents with his original body weight, that he had before his metabolic derangement had started. The elevated liver enzymes have normalized, the incipient type 2 diabetes has vanished, and also the lipid profile has nearly normalized. Fatty liver is no longer detectable by ultrasound.

Comment on Bruce K.

Patient Bruce K. (age 49) presents with signs of an early type 2 diabetes, lipid abnormalities, and fatty liver disease that taken together are central features of the metabolic syndrome. He also suffers from fatigue, physical exhaustion and a lack of concentration. The metabolic syndrome can largely be explained by a significant weight gain over the last 18 months and decreased physical activity and fitness. His PCP interprets these findings as symptoms of depression. Taking a closer history, we learn that Bruce has a family history of type 2 diabetes that affected both grandmothers. This points to a genetic predisposition that is well established for type 2 diabetes. Patients with type 2 diabetes are usually overweight, which goes along with inflammation of adipose tissues and frequently also with fatty liver inflammation (NASH). NASH has become the most common chronic liver disease in most countries of the world. Severe cases of NASH can lead to liver cirrhosis, liver failure, and liver cancer. Patients with type 2 diabetes, who are usually obese, carry a high risk to develop fatty liver disease, and NASH. Our preclinical studies show that ATI from foods promote obesity, type 2 diabetes and NASH. We can confirm this finding in the patients we see in our clinic. Currently, we have initiated a clinical study comparing a normal, wheat-based diet with the ATI-reduced diet in patients with fatty liver disease and incipient or manifest type 2 diabetes. The case of Bruce illustrates that an already advanced metabolic derangement improves shortly after the start of the ATI-reduced diet. After less than a year, the patient returns to his normal weight and regains his original constitution and fitness. It is evident that the ATI-reduced diet can also lead to reduced overall consumption of carbohydrate-containing foods, as many patients report. The weight loss that we observe in these patients is therefore certainly a combination of the ATI-reduction and a concomitant natural reduction of carbohydrate consumption. However, our research clearly shows that the avoidance of ATI alone has a significant effect on reducing symptoms of metabolic syndrome. This is also demonstrated for Bruce since his general condition starts to improve shortly after the dietary change.

5.8.5   Patient Kathy S. (40 Years): Food Allergies

Kathy S. is a 40-year-old patient who has experienced food-dependent symptoms for her whole life. She does not recall any longer periods in her life that were not dominated by abdominal pain, nausea, and frequent and watery bowel movements. In the last 3 years, these symptoms have worsened, and she felt that she was not able to cope with them anymore. She is a patient of a large GI practice, where numerous diagnostic studies had been performed, including regular blood tests, three upper endoscopies and two colonoscopies in the last 2 years alone. Breath tests for sugar intolerances had been carried out. Lactose intolerance was excluded, while a mild fructose intolerance was shown, a frequent finding in patients as well as healthy people that therefore is of limited clinical relevance. In addition, a blood test for IgE antibodies as well as a skin test for common food allergens yielded negative results. Based on the overall negative findings, her gastroenterologists arrived at the diagnosis of irritable bowel syndrome—a diagnosis of exclusion when no inflammatory disease is found. Accordingly, the therapeutic recommendations are relatively unspecific, such as: eat and live regularly and avoid coffee, spices, and stress. When she followed these recommendations, her condition did neither improve nor worsen. As before, Kathy complained about abdominal pain, frequent bowel movements up to five times a day, and diarrhea. A natural healer, whom she consulted in her despair, ordered an IgG blood test for food allergies. This test is not covered by health insurance (for a good reason). The results were shocking since Kathy appeared to be allergic to almost everything edible. Indicated were allergies to soy, egg, pineapple, chicken, fish and shellfish, various spices, peanuts, legumes, hazelnuts and walnuts, sesame, almonds, milk, quinoa, corn, apple, pear, stone fruits, and more. Her natural healer advised her to strictly avoid these foods. For almost half a year, she tried to adhere to this recommendation and profoundly restricted her diet. Basically, her residual diet consisted of potatoes, rice, steamed vegetables, bananas, small amounts of beef, and whole grains, especially spelt. She prepared everything herself to maintain control over the ingredients. To continue her social life, she even brought her own food to dinner invitations and restaurants. Although the complaints improved with this highly restricted diet, this regimen turned out to be not doable in the long run, especially since the already slim patient has lost another 6 kg (13.2 lb) in the last year and is now severely underweight (BMI 16.5). When Kathy presents in our clinic, she feels thoroughly exhausted and is in despair about her nutritional mess.

Our most important recommendation is to eliminate all ATI-containing foods, including spelt, and then to gradually reintroduce all previously "forbidden" foods in her diet again. For specification, she receives a dietary consult. Kathy, who lives 300 miles away, is allowed to stay in contact with us via email. Three weeks later, she reports that she has reintroduced several supposedly harmful foods step by step, i.e., every 2–3 days. First, she experiences some fear and resistance, but finally, when she realizes that she tolerates them well, with increasing confidence. Her postprandial belly pain and diarrhea, as well as her nausea, have almost resolved. The ATI-reduced diet is easy for her to follow. We recommend an additional intake of probiotics during this period of dietary readjustment. These are useful intestinal bacteria that can be taken in the form of capsules or chewable tablets. The patient receives two different probiotics, one for the microbial flora of the small intestine, one for the flora of the colon. After 4 weeks, the probiotics can be discontinued, since she is free of any complaints. Moreover, she has regained much of her former energy and of her original body weight with a BMI of 19. Kathy is now able to eat almost any food, except for soy and milk that she clearly identified as the cause for her abdominal discomfort.

Comment on Kathy S.
The 40-year-old patient Kathy S. complains of food-dependent abdominal pain, diarrhea, and nausea. Her gastroenterologists performed a battery of studies and didn't find a cause, leading to the diagnosis of irritable bowel syndrome (IBS). IBS is a diagnosis of exclusion that is often given when classical inflammatory diseases, including allergies, have been ruled out. The current hypothesis is that IBS is caused by nervous dysregulation in the gut and miscommunication between the brain and the gut. This is supposed to lead to a disturbance of the autonomous bowel movements to cause diarrhea or constipation, sometimes both alternately. Some patients report a severe intestinal infection before their symptoms began, and it is plausible that this may have led to a temporary or long-lasting disturbance of the intestinal motility. Psychological factors, such as stress, tension, and anxiety, can play a contributory role, but in our view, they are not the key pathologies. Accordingly, psychological or psychosomatic therapies have only limited efficacy in the treatment of IBS. In two recent studies, we have shown that a large proportion, up to 70%, of patients with IBS have an underlying food allergy that cannot be verified by the usual tests and methodologies, i.e., skin and IgE blood tests. Thus, the classical food allergy tests are negative for Kathy. A natural healer advised her to have an alternative blood test done, the so-called IgG test for allergies. However, these commercially offered "tests for food allergies" that are not reimbursed by healthcare providers are not of much help, but rather misleading. As in the case of Kathy, they often lead to extremely restricted diets, although the patient does not have an allergy

against the positively tested foods. An increased value merely indicates that individual components of these foods are resorbed by the intestine and recognized by the immune system. However, this immune recognition, as is shown by the positive IgG-antibodies, rather indicates protection than allergic sensitization, since they usually mirror a tolerance-inducing immune reaction that suppresses allergies and inflammation, instead of promoting them. This is precisely the normal immune reaction of the gut whose task it is to resorb foreign substances, the foodstuffs, not to fight them. It is exactly this reaction of active immune tolerance that the IgG blood test usually reflects. It is not a suitable tool to detect and define any form of allergy.

The patient had a large number of positive results. Since we do not interpret the positive results as an indication of an allergy, we recommend abandoning the extremely restricted diet that has already led to considerable physical and psychological harm. In fact, this strategy does not have any negative consequences for Kathy, as in most other patients. Nonetheless, it is possible and even likely that Kathy has an atypical food allergy that cannot be confirmed by current methods of testing. By using the special technology of confocal laser-endomicroscopy (CLE), we have identified wheat, milk, soy, and yeast, more rarely egg and nuts, as major foods that cause intestinal allergies. Notably, these are staples that almost everybody consumes daily and that are present in many refined foods. To date, such atypical allergies are difficult to prove, since this requires a complicated procedure with endoscopic food challenges followed by CLE that can only be done in a small number of patients within clinical studies and with substantial effort. Unfortunately, this technology is not available as a routine procedure.

For the treatment of Kathy's suspected food allergy, we furthermore suggest that she starts the ATI-reduced diet. This recommendation is based on our findings that nutritional and respiratory allergies are worsened by nutritional ATI. Therefore, she has to abandon spelt that she thought was particularly natural and healthy, but that is one of the major gluten and ATI-containing grains. She then is instructed to reintroduce every 2–3 days one of the foods that she had avoided before. With this regimen, she is doing well and discovers a severe reaction only to milk and soy that from now on she excludes from her diet. Under this far less restricted diet, Kathy's symptoms improve significantly within only a few weeks. Milk and soy are the second and third most frequent food allergens in patients with IBS. Importantly, wheat and related grains account for 60% of the atypical food allergies in IBS. Adhering to the ATI-reduced diet, therefore, in a way automatically eliminates wheat and related grains as major food allergens. In Kathy's case, both mechanisms may play a role, ATI as promoters of her soy and milk allergy, plus ATI-containing grains as allergens themselves.

5.8.6   Patient Laura K. (23 Years): Persistent Skin Eczema

The 23-year-old patient Laura K. is a law student in her third year. She complains of waxing and waning skin eczema since age 15. The eczema is prominent on the palms of both hands. The affected skin is dry and red with occasional blisters, painful cracks, and severe itching. Sometimes it spreads to the forearms and even to her thighs. Recently, it has also erupted on her face, especially around her nostrils and the corners of her mouth. During these episodes, Laura is particularly tormented by the itching and her "disfigurement", especially as the wet blisters around her nose cannot be concealed. Laura also fears that this leads to permanent disfiguration of her face. She has been treated by a dermatologist for many years. Allergies were excluded, and no triggers could be identified in the household or in everyday life, such as ingredients in detergents, cosmetics, or soaps. Therefore, she was diagnosed with endogenous eczema, i.e., eczema without an identified cause. She has always meticulously followed the advice regarding basic measures of handwashing and facial care and strictly avoided contact with irritating substances. Laura also uses several prescribed ointments and lotions that at best provide some relief. She has also used topical cortisone and ointments with the immunosuppressive agent Tacrolimus that are quite effective. However, these immunosuppressants can only be used for a few weeks due to their unwanted side effects. Two months ago, Laura attended a seminar in a monastery with meditation and fasting. To her surprise, her entire eczema improved dramatically, with only minor skin changes remaining on her palms. Back home in everyday life, dominated by her classes, homework, and her job, as well as a resumption of her normal diet, her eczema has returned even worse than before. She presents in our outpatient clinic asking how far her diet may underlie her skin disease and tells us that during fasting, she became symptom-free for the first time in 8 years. During fasting, she had lived exclusively on tea and vegetable broth. Her extensive medical records reveal that a repetitive series of allergy tests had been performed—both skin and blood tests—all with negative results.

As with our prior patient Kathy S., we discover in her records the well-known IgG test for food allergens. Laura's IgG results show increased levels for pineapple, stone fruits, milk, and eggs. Therefore, she has been avoiding these foods for the last 2 years. In addition, there are findings from various stool tests showing an increase in Candida fungi and a reduction in supposedly useful bacteria, namely lactobacilli and bifidobacteria. Based on the Candida results, her PCP repeatedly advised her to take an antifungal for several weeks. But she refused this medication for fear of considerable side effects.

Like in Kathy S.'s case we recommend that Laura ignores the IgG tests for food allergens and that she starts to eat dairy products again since the lack of milk in her diet alone explains the unfavorable counts of the useful lactobacilli and bifidobacteria in her stool samples. We assure her that she had been right to reject the antifungal drug because there is no evidence for a pathogenic role of stool Candida fungi in patients with a normal immune system. Antifungal therapies can have considerable side effects and are only useful for patients with a severe, clearly defined fungal infection, usually patients with a severe immune defect. There is no medical indication to use them to eradicate naturally occurring intestinal fungi.

Laura presents with a typical so-called endogenous eczema. The term "endogenous" is generally used when no definable cause of a disease is found. Taking our usual in-depth history, it becomes clear that it was her fasting diet in the monastery that led to the cure of her eczema. This diet contained only vegetable broth and herbal tea, and no bread for 7 days. Notably, bread and other wheat products are the major allergens in more than 60% of patients with atypical "allergens" including endogenous eczema. Therefore, for now, our only recommendation to Laura is to pursue the wheat and ATI-reduced diet and to continue with her otherwise balanced nutrition. We see her again after 4 weeks. Her facial eczema has almost disappeared, as has her palmar eczema. After another 3 months, she presents to inform us that for the first time in 8 years she has remained completely symptom-free.

Comment on Laura K.

Laura K. (23 years) complains of a therapy-resistant skin eczema. While this is reminiscent of an allergy in a broader sense, no allergen has been found with conventional testing—hence the name "endogenous". Current understanding incriminates genetic, psychological, and environmental factors to cause the disease. However, none of these ill-defined factors has led to a clue how to treat or cure the condition specifically. Current treatments, including strong immunosuppressive drugs, only alleviate the symptoms.

Our research findings from animal experiments clearly demonstrate that wheat proteins are primary food allergens (see Chap. 7) and, additionally, that ATI promote allergies in general. Since endogenous eczema shows disease mechanism of allergies, we can conclude that Laura's eczema may respond to the wheat- and ATI-reduced diet alone. In fact, Laura reports that her eczema had almost disappeared with the fasting diet in the monastery. However, patients cannot fast for life. Here the ATI-reduced diet is an educated first-line recommendation with a high chance of success. In Laura's case, this measure was more effective than any other prior drug treatment, including topical immunosuppressants like cortisone and Tacrolimus.

Laura's case also shows that the widespread belief that endogenous eczema is prominently induced by psychological stress and thus more a psychosomatic than a somatic disease cannot be upheld. Thus, her symptoms improved dramatically, although the resumed her stressful schedule. Moreover, she expanded her dietary choices, including IgG-positive foods.

Whether Laura represents a case of a hidden wheat allergy or another allergy that is intensified by ATI, cannot be answered conclusively. An endoscopic provocation using CLE would be necessary for differential diagnosis (see Chap. 7). Practically, this does not make any difference for Laura.

5.8.7   Patient William P. (63 Years): Rheumatoid Arthritis

William P. (63) is a branch manager of a savings bank and is looking forward to his retirement at age 65. He has been a widow for 5 years and has a daughter who lives with her family of two children in a separate apartment of his house. She often asks her father to join for family meals. However, William is increasingly occupied with his chronic disease and is worried that he will not be able to enjoy his retirement. William has to cope with joint swelling and joint pain for 20 years, especially at the metacarpophalangeal joints of both hands, the wrists and both elbows. He also deals with increasing generalized muscle and joint pain and physical exhaustion. 18 years ago he was diagnosed with rheumatoid arthritis. Since then, he has received numerous therapies, initially with so-called basic therapeutics or disease-modifying antirheumatic drugs (DMARDs), namely gold salts, 5-ASA (aminosalicylic acid) and Chloroquine. During episodes of acute worsening, he frequently had to take high doses of cortisone for several weeks. With these treatments, the disease had largely been under control. In the last 6 years, he has received injections of antibodies against the body's own inflammatory cytokine, TNF-alpha, every 2–4 weeks, after discontinuing the DMARDs that did not work anymore. With the TNF-alpha therapy, the disease progression has stabilized, although he still needs painkillers to be able to lead his daily life. X-ray images show worsening of the affected joints and bones. William also perceives his disease as disfiguring, and he has increasing difficulties to write and to perform smaller manual tasks such as repairing and assembling. He has noticed a reduced strength in both hands, making it difficult for him even to put on stockings or open a jam jar. Williams rheumatologist recommends resuming regular exercise despite his pain. However, his 30-min-fitness program that his physiotherapist designed for him has become an ordeal. His rheumatologist, therefore, decided to discontinue the TNF-alpha antibody therapy and prescribes another antibody, targeting activated T cells. When we see him, he has received these injections for 4 months. He has noticed a minor improvement of pain and motility, but also side effects such as dizziness and nausea. His body weight is in the normal range and his diet is diversified and balanced, but he has a soft spot for handmade cookies from his local bakery. His daughter, who persuaded him to see us and accompanies him, tells us that she is worried about her father's loss of energy and capabilities. She has read about nutrition and chronic diseases and that a gluten-free diet might be beneficial for her father, also in view of his "addiction" to his favorite cookies. He considers the gluten-free diet as a fad and has come to our clinic only to do his daughter a favor.

Physical examination confirms moderately advanced rheumatoid arthritis. Blood levels of inflammation markers—rheumatoid factor, CRP (C-reactive protein) and CCP (cyclic citrullinated peptide) antibodies—are mildly elevated. The metacarpophalangeal joints are visibly swollen, the hands show the typical ulnar deviation and William reports impairment and pain when using his hands. After the 4 months of treatment with the novel antibody that only led to a mild improvement, but also to side effects, he has lost trust in novel therapies. We explain the role of ATI in inflammatory diseases, even inflammatory diseases outside the intestine. We succeed to convince him that his disease might be driven by his ATI/wheat consumption. He finally agrees to start the ATI-reduced diet for a trial period of 4 weeks. His daughter assures us to support her father and to make sure that he will be able to follow the dietary guidelines of the ATI-reduced diet, namely, to omit all obvious wheat/gluten-containing foods. This rule will lead to a 95% reduction of ATI in the daily diet, sufficient not to cause disease since the ATI effect is dose-dependent.

After 4 weeks, we see the patient again. He has tried to follow the diet with his daughter's help, but admits to have had three glitches having bought some cookies from his favorite bakery during lunch breaks. Nonetheless, he reports a felt improvement of his joint pain, general condition, and performance. His morning exercise has changed from "ordeal to cumbersome duty". Still, he is not entirely convinced that the ATI-reduced diet has brought about the change, since he recalls such periods of spontaneous improvement in the past. But he considers it worthwhile to continue the diet for another month, this time more strictly. We see him after another 8 weeks. William now describes an undoubted improvement of his joint pains and general condition. The blood test shows a decrease in the inflammation markers. He hasn't taken any other medication except for some pain killers and the monthly T cell antibodies, and this time he has strictly complied with the ATI-reduced diet. He now consumes only gluten/ATI-free pastries and is not craving anymore for his favorite cookies. Now he is convinced and motivated to continue the ATI-reduced diet long-term, also because he has lost 2 kg of body weight, which further increased his motivation to exercise more. When we see William 1 year after the start of the ATI-reduced diet, he is still in remission, i.e., his disease is well under control, now with the T cell antibody being given only once in 3 months. He does not need regular pain killers anymore. His general condition is greatly improved, and he is looking forward to an active retirement.

Comment on William P.
William P. (63 years) suffers from a chronic inflammatory disease of the joints, rheumatoid arthritis. Rheumatoid arthritis is an autoimmune disease in which the body's own T cells fight against the connective tissue of the joints. The causes of rheumatoid arthritis are complex. There is a genetic predisposition as well as ill-defined additional environmental influences, for example, infections or stressful life events. The disease usually affects the metacarpophalangeal joints, but also other joints and soft tissues of the body. Rheumatoid arthritis is a systemic disease. The patients feel fatigued, weakened, and impaired in their overall performance. Because of the pain, especially during movement, there is a risk of inactivity and subsequent immobilization. Inactivity further drives the loss of function of important joints, such as in hands and knees. If not instructed appropriately, patients increasingly avoid movement, which starts a vicious circle of pain and immobility. There is a plethora of drugs, the so-called "basic therapeutics" (DMARDs), that are used to treat less severe cases in the long term. Many patients, however, need stronger medicines, such as cortisone and other immune-suppressive drugs, including biologicals. The biologicals are mostly antibodies against the body's own inflammatory cells or cytokines that are given at intervals ranging from once weekly to once every 2–3 months. William has received DMARDs from the start of his disease 18 years ago, periodically combined with cortisone. A biological, a TNF-alpha antibody, was started 6 years ago. When the TNF-alpha antibody lost efficacy, William was changed over to another biological, a T cell blocking antibody. However, despite the escalated therapy, his general condition continually worsened. This is the situation when we see him the first time. He feels hopeless and disillusioned, and he only presents, because his daughter insisted. She has read about dietary management of rheumatoid arthritis, including a gluten-free diet, but William is unconvinced and

believes this is a mere fad. We educate both that there is indeed a solid scientific basis for the ATI-reduced diet in rheumatoid arthritis, as in other autoimmune diseases. With this scientific evidence, we can overcome William's resistance, and he agrees to give it a try for 4 weeks. Except for his minor dietary transgressions, he keeps with the diet and reports a significant improvement that motivates him to go on, even more diet-adherent than before. After another 2 months of the ATI-reduced diet pain and immobility have improved and this continues for another year, the last time that we see him. At this time, he receives his T cell antibody as maintenance therapy only every 3 months instead of once a month before. His previously elevated markers of inflammation have normalized or near normalized. This case is another example that the ATI-reduced diet usually leads to a significant improvement of an autoimmune disease. Obviously, William has needed several weeks until he experiences a significant improvement in his joint symptoms. In this case, there is a delayed onset of the improvement, because rheumatoid arthritis is a complex chronic inflammatory disease that involves the whole body's immune system and particularly the connective tissues of joints, tendons, bones, and muscles. Understandably, more extended periods of time are needed for the reversal of the pathological processes. However, William's general condition has improved within 4 weeks, which has been a strong motivation to continue with the ATI-reduced diet and other lifestyle changes long-term.

5.8.8 Summary of the Cases with ATI-Sensitivity

The presented cases cover much of the broad clinical spectrum of ATI-sensitivity. ATI-sensitivity worsens pre-existing chronic conditions, such as auto-immune, but also cardiovascular and metabolic diseases, including type 2 diabetes and fatty liver inflammation. It is even likely that ATI do not only exacerbate, but also promote the first manifestation of these conditions. It is still unclear whether a certain genetic predisposition makes certain people more susceptible to the effects of nutritional ATI. ATI are important, but not the only responsible co-factors for chronic inflammatory diseases, because there are also other influences, such as infections, side effects of drugs, intestinal dysbiosis due to antibiotics and more. The ATI-reduced diet is usually surprisingly effective, even more effective than most medications. We can explain this efficiency by the ATI's dual effect of activating innate immunity and inducing intestinal dysbiosis. Notably, the ATI-reduced diet is relatively easy to follow. First, it is largely identical to the gluten-free diet; second, minor amounts of ATI do not cause harm and do not have to be strictly avoided (different from gluten in celiac disease). Our definition of the ATI-reduced diet is as follows: We recommend that the daily ATI consumption should be below 5% of the standard "Western" diet. The Western diet usually includes 120–200 g wheat flour, 15–25 g of gluten and 0.7–1.2 g of ATI. The ATI-reduced diet can easily be carried out just by omitting obvious ATI-containing foods like bread, pizza, or pasta.

Chapter 6
Lactose, Fructose and Histamine Intolerance: Over-Diagnosed and Overrated

We have included this chapter since patients who present to us with food-related complaints often have been diagnosed with lactose, fructose, or histamine intolerance before. Importantly, fructose and lactose intolerances do not cause any inflammation and therefore, no harm. Patients might experience a mild improvement of their symptoms, especially bloating, on the respective diets, but often continue to have severe symptoms. In the beginning, the treating physicians are usually happy to have made a diagnosis that might lead to some benefit. Since severe symptoms usually persist in the longer run, patients often resort to extreme and unhealthy diets, such as the complete exclusion of fruits and vegetables, in order to avoid fructose or histamine. In fact, these patients frequently have one of the inflammatory food diseases, such as celiac disease, and more often ATI-sensitivity or atypical allergies, primarily against wheat, as described in Chap. 7.

In our practice as in general, patients with abdominal discomfort and symptoms of a suspected food intolerance frequently present with a diagnosis of fructose, lactose, or histamine intolerance based on prior laboratory testing. These intolerances can indeed lead to bloating and some abdominal pain. Importantly, patients with mere sugar (fructose and lactose) intolerance do not have signs of intestinal inflammation (see Chap. 5). Fructose and lactose are essential constituents of FODMAPs, i.e., foods that can cause bloating and diarrhea, but are non-inflammatory and harmless (see Sect. 5.7.10; FODMAP = fermentable oligo-, di-, monosaccharides, and polyols). Therefore, we use the term intolerance, in contrast to sensitivity—the latter term is reserved for inflammatory processes. Symptoms of these sugar intolerances result from their reduced uptake via the intestinal mucosa and therefore an increased bacterial fermentation of the sugar remaining in the intestine. To repeat: This does not go along with inflammation.

© Springer Nature Switzerland AG 2019
D. Schuppan, K. Gisbert-Schuppan, *Wheat Syndromes*
https://doi.org/10.1007/978-3-030-19023-1_6

6.1   Lactose Intolerance

There is a genetic basis for lactose intolerance. Those affected lack an enzyme in the intestinal mucosa, lactase, which breaks down the milk sugar lactose. Chemically, lactose is a dimeric sugar, which is broken down by lactase into its single sugars glucose and galactose. Only these monomeric sugars can be absorbed by the intestinal epithelium. If lactase is missing from the intestinal epithelium, the dimeric lactose remains in the intestine and is fermented by the intestinal bacteria producing gas. This leads to bloating, but can also cause diarrhea, since the sugar is osmotically active in the intestine, i.e., the unfermented sugar draws water into the intestine. These mechanisms explain the symptoms of the patients: bloating and diarrhea. However, there is a broad spectrum of complaints among those patients. Some are very sensitive and react to small amounts of lactose; others can tolerate modest or even moderate amounts. Dairy products produced by lactobacilli or certain fungi (kefir), that ferment of much of the lactose to lactic acid are better tolerated than fresh milk products. Patients can also use lactase as enzyme supplement and food additive that will split the dimeric lactose to glucose and galactose. We recommend that patients with lactose intolerance consume smaller amounts of dairy products, as tolerated, since lactobacilli belong to the favorable intestinal bacteria, but they only thrive if they can feed on dairy products. Even without laboratory testing, most people affected already know that they do not tolerate fresh dairy products. A breath test can confirm lactose intolerance. The patient drinks a solution of lactose, and in the following 2 h the exhaled hydrogen concentration is determined. An increased exhaled hydrogen value indicates bacterial fermentation in the intestine and thus lactose intolerance. During this challenge, the lactose intolerant person also reports abdominal discomfort. Recently, a genetic test has been developed that is becoming more frequently used. In this test, blood cells that contain all the genetic information of the body, and therefore also the lactase gene, are tested for the presence of the non-functional variant. The lactase genotype-1 is the most frequently occurring non-functional variant worldwide. Interestingly, the other variant that remains active up to old age has only become dominant in populations that practiced livestock breeding and continued to consume cow's milk beyond infancy –like in the Western world. After birth, all infants worldwide are equipped with the functioning enzyme, in order to digest the mother's breast milk, but usually lose it during early childhood and become lactose intolerant, as is found in most inhabitants of Southeast Asia and East Asia today.

6.2   Fructose Intolerance

Fructose intolerance is diagnosed all too often.[1] Fructose is an essential part of our diet and occurs naturally in fruits and vegetables. Fructose intolerance is not based on a genetic mutation like lactose intolerance, although symptoms are similar.

---

[1] In the extremely rare condition of "Genetic Fructose Intolerance" that must be taken very seriously the body lacks an enzyme, fructaldolase, that leads to the accumulation of a toxic metabolic

Larger amounts of fructose are not completely absorbed by the intestinal mucosa. Like in lactose intolerance, the excess fructose remains in the intestine for a prolonged time causing bloating and abdominal pain by bacterial fermentation and sometimes inducing diarrhea by an increased influx of water into the intestine. Fructose intolerance is essentially a problem of quantity. With the modern Western diet, we all consume excessive amounts of fructose, since fructose is added to most processed foods as a cheap sweetener. These large quantities overload the fructose transporter on the intestinal epithelial cells, while there are individual differences in the fructose uptake capacity. Interestingly, fructose is better absorbed if it is consumed in approximately the same concentration as glucose, as there is a glucose-fructose co-transport across the intestinal epithelium. Even in case the fructose breath test, which is similar to the lactose breath test, indicates fructose intolerance, this does not mean that fructose must be entirely avoided. Those with a positive breath test or suspected fructose intolerance should individually find out how much fructose or what fruits and vegetables they tolerate best. Information about fructose content and tolerability of foods is also available on the internet.

6.3 Histamine Intolerance

Symptoms of histamine intolerance appear immediately after the meal and can manifest as redness, swelling, and itching of the skin and mucous membranes, headaches, dizziness, asthma, runny nose, tachycardia and also abdominal discomfort such as bloating, diarrhea, constipation, nausea, vomiting, pain, and heartburn. Histamine intolerance is still considered a controversial food intolerance, and some researcher and physicians doubt that it even exists. But there is sufficient evidence that some patients indeed are histamine intolerant. Histamine is a so-called biogenic amine, a degradation product of the naturally occurring and essential amino acid histidine. Histamine is a central messenger in allergies. It is released from the body's mast cells when the allergen-specific IgE antibodies have bound to their allergen. Histamine released in the allergic reaction is a central mediator of the known allergy symptoms that include the contraction of the respiratory muscles causing asthma, and dilatation of the blood vessels of the mucous membranes causing their swelling, inflammation and fluid secretion. Histamine is also found in a number of foods. Histamine rich foods are seafood smoked meats such as certain sausages and ham, offal such as liver and kidney, cheese, particularly mature cheeses, pickled foods like sauerkraut, red wine, beer, ketchup, strawberries, and tomatoes. Normally, food-derived histamine is broken down effectively by the body's own enzymes. These are diamine oxidase (DAO) that destroys histamine by oxidation and histamine-N-methyltransferase (HNMT) that inactivates histamine by methylation

---

product, fructose-1-phosphate, in the intestine and liver. An even rarer genetic enzyme defect is fructose-1,6-phosphatase deficiency. These 2 genetic diseases are usually diagnosed in early infancy. Therefore, those affected know about their condition. The severe intolerances are of course excluded from our explanations in this chapter.

and promotes its excretion via the kidneys. DAO is often determined in the blood, but blood levels hardly reflect tissue levels or show how far the enzyme is active or not. However, an extremely low DAO level can be an indication of histamine intolerance. At the same time, a normal DAO level does not exclude histamine intolerance. The level of HNMT in a 24-hour urine sample is probably more indicative, as it correlates with increased exposure to histamine that has not been inactivated by DAO. Histamine is absorbed by the intestine and can cause typical symptoms of food allergy with abdominal as well as peripheral signs. The internet provides helpful classifications of histamine-rich foods. Practically, the diagnosis of histamine intolerance is straight forward, since patients report an improvement of their symptoms simply by avoiding histamine containing foods. For patients, it is also comforting to know that histamine intolerance can fluctuate across the lifespan.

6.4 Summary

Taken together, we often see patients with a diagnosis of lactose, fructose or histamine intolerance and no improvement on the respective diet. Usually, these patients have a different underlying condition, especially wheat induced sensitivities: celiac disease, ATI-sensitivity or (atypical) allergies. Except for celiac disease, these inflammatory diseases cannot be diagnosed by current laboratory tests or endoscopic procedures, and therefore are not recognized by physicians. Therefore, doctors tend to attribute patients' complaints to one of the three discussed food intolerances once one of the tests has turned out positive. To the patients' despair, the symptoms often do not improve since the intolerance tests have been misleading. Following their doctor's advice or their own interpretation of the positive test results, they often completely avoid dairy products, fruits, and vegetables, or the many potential sources of histamine, without much improvement. This often leads to severe dietary restrictions and a deficiency in valuable nutrients. We encourage patients diagnosed with lactose, fructose (and somewhat more carefully) with histamine intolerance to find out for themselves how much of these foods they tolerate well since they cannot do anything substantially wrong in testing them out. After all, the sugar intolerances are non-inflammatory conditions, not comparable to the inflammatory sensitivities. Histamine intolerance can be seen as an exception since some forms of severe histamine intolerance (even with signs of anaphylactic shock) have been reported. We want to stress that patients often have other underlying, inflammatory food sensitivities that are neglected and overlooked by concentrating on the sugar intolerances that we have discussed in this chapter.

Chapter 7
Classical and Atypical Food Allergies

In this chapter, symptoms of classical food allergies with immediate reactions are described first. Skin and IgE blood tests for classical food allergens have some but limited diagnostic value. IgG blood tests are no useful diagnostic tools. In this chapter, we also introduce atypical food allergies as a new entity. They are IgE blood test and skin test negative. The atypical allergies are more frequent than the classical allergies, and their diagnosis is difficult since symptoms usually occur with a delay of several hours after allergen ingestion. Major atypical allergens are wheat, followed by milk, soy, and yeast. These allergies can be diagnosed with a novel endoscopic method. They account for approximately 70% of patients with a previous diagnosis of irritable bowel syndrome. Three extensively commented clinical cases from our own practice round-up this chapter.

7.1 Introduction to Classical and Atypical Food Allergies

The symptoms of classical food allergies resemble those of commonly known allergies, such as allergic asthma or allergies due to insect bites. Their feature is an immediate reaction with acute symptoms like shortness of breath, cough, a runny nose and redness, swelling and itching of the skin, lips, palate, nasal mucous membranes and eyes. These reactions can become life-threatening, and patients may need emergency treatment. The triggers of classical allergies are usually relatively easy to identify. In most food allergies, however, identifying the allergen can be difficult, even more so in the newly discovered and described atypical allergies. These atypical allergies are more prevalent than the classical allergies characterized by a noticeable immediate reaction to food. Insidiously, in atypical food allergy symptoms occur with a delay, usually after several hours. Symptoms primarily affect the gastrointestinal tract and are mainly abdominal pain, bloating, diarrhea, and also constipation. A positive diagnosis can only be obtained by a novel endoscopic technique (see below). For this reason, these food reactions have not been recognized as

© Springer Nature Switzerland AG 2019
D. Schuppan, K. Gisbert-Schuppan, *Wheat Syndromes*
https://doi.org/10.1007/978-3-030-19023-1_7

Typical food allergens

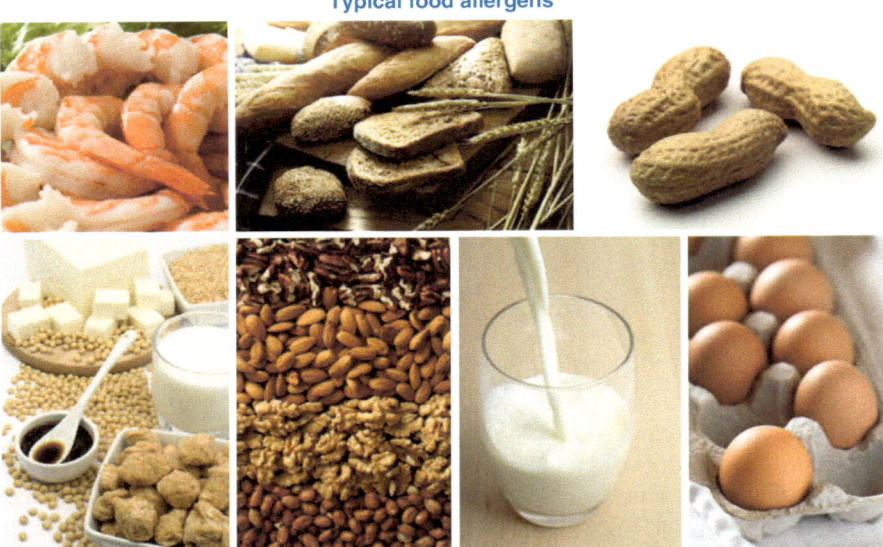

Fig. 7.1 The most relevant food allergens. Classical (IgE-mediated) food allergies are more frequent in children (4–6%) than in adults (1–4%). In contrast, atypical (IgE and skin test negative) food allergies are very common, and found in an estimated 5–10% of adults. Currently, these atypical allergies cannot be confirmed with conventional tests, but require a special endoscopic diagnostic procedure. Moreover, symptoms, mainly abdominal pain, bloating, diarrhea or constipation, kick in with a delay of up to several hours after consumption of the causative food allergens (mainly wheat (60%), followed by yeast, milk and soy)

allergies for a long time, and many of the patients receive the label "irritable bowel syndrome". The most frequent food allergens are shown in Fig. 7.1.

7.2 Even Classical Food Allergies can be Difficult to Diagnose

Approved tests for food and pollen allergies measure IgE antibodies against allergens. Allergic patients often, but not always, display increased blood levels of these IgE antibodies. High titer IgE antibodies to a given allergen are indeed indicative of an allergy, for example, to specific pollen, house dust mites, and also to foods such as nuts, soy, milk protein, particular raw vegetable and fruits, seafood, or cereals like wheat or rye. The IgE antibodies, like other antibodies—such as IgG and IgA—are produced by B lymphocytes. The allergen-specific IgE antibodies bind to the allergen to form a complex. This complex is recognized by tissue mast cells,[1] another

---

[1] This includes mast cells and also basophilic and eosinophilic granulocytes.

class of immune cells. In evolution, mast cells have played an important role in the expulsion of parasites, since they secrete highly effective substances (mediators) that lead to the contraction of smooth muscle cells. Smooth muscle cells are found in the respiratory tract, the intestine, and in blood vessels, those organs that can contract vigorously in allergic reactions. These contractions make sense since they help to eliminate the invader, but they can become troublesome and sometimes life-threatening in case of allergies. Moreover, in allergic people, this reaction is directed against a normally harmless pollen or food antigen. The mechanism of IgE-mediated allergies is illustrated in Fig. 7.2. The question arises why do patients develop allergies towards normally harmless environmental antigens at all? It is also not clear why allergies in most populations have doubled in the last 20–30 years. A possible

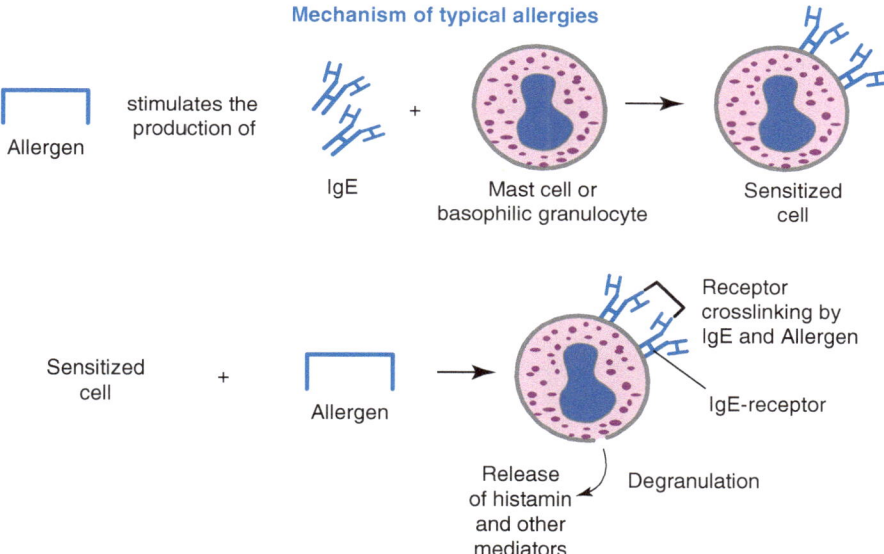

Fig. 7.2 Mechanisms of classical allergies. The allergen, usually a protein, initially induces the production of antibodies of the IgE class in specialized B lymphocytes. Mast cells and basophilic granulocytes carry receptors for IgE. The allergen-specific IgE binds to the IgE receptor and thus coats the surface of these cells. In case of a subsequent contact with the allergen via the mucosal membranes of the airways or the intestine (to a lesser degree via the skin) mast cells and basophils are then prepared to bind the allergen via the cell-bound, allergen-specific IgE. Two IgE molecules and two IgE-receptors need to be bound by a single allergen to trigger a signal in the mast cell or the basophil (receptor cross-linking). Each allergen must therefore have two IgE binding sites, in order to be effective. This is followed by an immediate release of histamine and other mediators that cause the typical symptoms of an allergy within only a few minutes, such as dilatation of blood vessels (flush), mucosal swelling (extravasation of plasma and infiltration of inflammatory cells into the tissue), shortness of breath, cramping or diarrhea (contraction of respiratory or gastrointestinal smooth muscle cells), itching and pain (inflammation and pain producing mediators). A hyposensitization is based on the careful induction of antibodies of the IgG class, mainly via subcutaneous or oral vaccination. These IgG antibodies do not bind to mast cells or basophils, but rather block the binding of the allergen to the cell-bound IgE

explanation is that societies where the prevalence of allergies is highest, the immune system has not learned to develop immune tolerance to potential allergens in early formative years. In this context, the hygiene hypothesis provides an explanation. It is based on the fact that the increase of allergies goes hand in hand with improved sanitation and hygiene. Less hygiene in early life confronts the organism with a wide variety of microbes. Only this way, the infant's immune system is educated to develop tolerance against harmless bacteria and likely allergens ("old friends" hypothesis). It is also conceivable that an overall change in the environment and therefore in the microbiome of the respiratory tract, the skin, and especially the intestine, has led to an increased susceptibility for allergies. This is likely connected to a change in eating habits, and here especially high consumption of refined foods that have replaced natural foods. Allergies are also promoted by the consumption of ATI in wheat and related grains. We have explained the mechanism of how this works on the cellular and molecular level. We also see this adjuvant effect of ATI, the general promotion of allergies, in our patients (see also Chap. 5).

7.3   Testing for Classical Food Allergy

In classical wheat allergy, as an example for classical food allergies, IgE antibodies against wheat proteins, including gluten, may be detectable in the blood. Some patients react to wheat or gluten in skin testing. Skin testing is performed by applying a small amount of the allergen to the skin via a tiny scratch or prick on the inside of the forearm. In case of an allergy, a small swelling with redness can develop. This is the so-called scratch or prick test. Allergens can also be applied with an adhesive patch—the patch test. Unfortunately, these allergen tests have a limited predictive value, i.e., the reaction is often negative, even when an allergy is present. Occasionally, there is a false positive reaction, too. Nonetheless, IgE and skin tests are helpful tools that can support the clinical diagnosis of a classical food allergy.

In contrast, the broadly offered and frequently used allergen screens, often recommended by non-expert healers, that are based on IgG antibodies are useless. They cover a wide spectrum of potential inhalative and food allergens. The production of IgG antibodies is elicited by numerous harmless food components that often enter the intestinal mucosa without triggering an allergy. Rather, these IgG antibodies can be considered protective antibodies as are induced during desensitization. In desensitization, small amounts of the allergen are administered to the patient subcutaneously or sublingually. The induced IgG antibodies against the allergen then block the complex formation between the allergen and IgE antibodies that are causing mast cell activation.

In our practice, we often see patients with food-dependent complaints who have elevated IgG antibodies against 10–20 foods. These patients, therefore, believe that they can hardly eat anything and subject themselves to a highly restricted and unhealthy diet. As a consequence, they can show signs of vitamin, mineral, and protein deficiencies that are otherwise rarely found with balanced nutrition. It takes some effort to convince these patients that they have to add the supposedly harmful foods back to their diet gradually. To the patients' surprise, they realize that they tolerate most of these foods very well. Examples of such allegedly "allergenic foods" are egg, pineapple, stone fruit, avocado, parsley, spinach, spices and many more. While these foods can be triggers of classical, IgE antibody positive allergies, the production of IgG antibodies rather indicates a state of active tolerance.

7.4   Most Food Allergies Remain Undetected: Atypical Allergies

7.4.1   What are Atypical Food Allergies?

Most patients with classical food allergies are IgE blood or skin test positive. The atypical allergies are very different. Their allergic symptoms are not immediate and arise 30 min to many hours after food intake. Patients report abdominal pain, bloating and diarrhea, sometimes also constipation or both in alternation. Standard endoscopy fails to detect inflammatory changes of the gastrointestinal tract, and symptoms cannot be easily connected with specific foods. Therefore, these patients receive the diagnosis of irritable bowel syndrome (IBS). So far, the IBS has mainly been attributed to physical or psychological stress, depression and/or post-infectious changes in the intestinal tract. Symptoms are also attributed to a disturbance of the autonomous intestinal as well as the central nervous system. IBS has significant implications for society and the health care system. According to recent studies, approximately 15% of Western populations and increasing numbers worldwide suffer from these symptoms. Apart from being a burden for the many patients, the disease leads to considerable absence from work and loss of productivity.

We clearly demonstrated that 70% of patients with a former IBS diagnosis improve markedly on a hypoallergenic diet, consisting of potatoes and/or rice, olive oil, and salt for three to 5 days. This improvement can only be explained by food as a trigger of symptoms instead of a primary dysregulation of the nervous systems. In our clinical studies, we have shown that the majority (another 70%) of the 70% food reactive patients display an immediate inflammatory reaction to four general foods in the upper small intestine. We call these foods the "Big Four": Wheat, milk, soy, and yeast. The remaining 30% is due to other foods than the Big Four. Thus, we have seen comparable reactions to nuts and eggs, and there will be rarer atypical allergens. The immediate mucosal reaction after intestinal allergen application (the procedure is described in detail in the following chapter) confirms that these patients do indeed have a food allergy. Just in 2019, we could publish an extensive clinical study that suggests a causative role of eosinophilic lymphocytes, in contrast to mast cells in classical allergies.

Importantly, patients become symptom-free after exclusion of the identified food allergen. The targeted exclusion diet is far more effective in the treatment of patients with a former IBS diagnosis than currently recommended untargeted diets, such as the low FODMAP diet. It is also far more effective than all medication that is on the market for IBS. In our studies, we also found that a substantial proportion the 30% of patients with an IBS diagnosis that do not improve on the hypoallergenic diet belong to another category. These patients have had a severe intestinal infection that might have damaged the intestinal nervous system and therefore, intestinal motility. These patients do no respond well to diets. Here the term "post-infectious IBS" is appropriate. Except for this special group, the unspecific term and the diagnosis of IBS needs to be replaced.

7.4.2   Diagnosis of Atypical Food Allergy

Together with our colleague Annette Fritscher-Ravens and her coworkers in London, UK, and Kiel, Germany, we have validated a novel endoscopic method to diagnose the atypical allergies. With her team, she has developed a methodology combining allergen provocation in the intestine with magnification endoscopy. The allergens are applied to the small intestine through the endoscope. Solutions or suspensions of four common foods were sprayed on the intestinal mucosa at 5-min intervals from distal to proximal. The magnification endoscope, the so-called confocal laser endo-microscope, allows the recording of mucosal changes with a 1000-fold magnification. With this technology, allergy-typical immediate reactions on the mucosa can be observed that otherwise would have remained undetected. The major allergens that lead to such acute allergic reactions in the intestine are the "Big Four": wheat, milk, soy, and yeast. Other food allergens that play a role in classical, IgE or skin test positive allergies, like egg and nuts, rarely cause such reactions. In our first study, we found that 22 out of 32 IBS patients with food-dependent symptoms showed an immediate inflammatory reaction of the mucosa, i.e., an increased infiltration of inflammatory cells, an opening of the tight junctions that connect the epithelial cells, a shedding of the epithelial cells into the lumen, a mucosal edema and, as a hallmark, exudation of tissue fluid into the gut lumen. To make the inflammatory changes visible through the endoscope, the patients receive a prior intravenous injection of a harmless fluorescent dye. Notably, 13 of the 22 study patients with an immediate response reacted to wheat. We recently confirmed these results in a much larger study of 106 food sensitive patients with a former IBS diagnosis. This study showed again that 2 thirds of them react to one of the allergens of the Big Four, rarely to egg or nuts, and that 60% reacted to wheat. If we extrapolate these data, assuming that 15% of the population has to deal with the symptoms of IBS, we predict that at least 7–8% of the overall population will have an undetected, atypical allergy to one of the tested foods and that up to 4% of the population will have an atypical allergy to wheat. These numbers illustrate the enormous implications of atypical food allergies for the health care system, the whole population and, prominently, the so-called IBS patients, of whom in fact the majority have atypical food allergies.

Some study patients reacted not only to 1 but 2 of the applied 4 allergens. Again, patients usually reported abdominal symptoms after several hours up to 24 h after the challenge. This is a major reason why identification of the allergenic food is difficult, if not impossible for the affected patients themselves. This is the more remarkable, since the mucosal reaction, as was observed via the endo-microscope, became apparent within 5 min. To obtain insight into the underlying mechanism of the atypical allergies, we took duodenal biopsy samples before and after the food challenge. As expected and as is the rule for patients with the diagnosis of IBS, these biopsies did not reveal significant pathological changes according to standard criteria, except for mildly increased intraepithelial lymphocytes, i.e., very mild inflammation that can also be found in some normal healthy control patients. Such a finding would usually have confirmed the standard diagnosis IBS, suggesting the lack of an inflammatory reaction. Only with refined immunological analysis of the same biopsies after challenge, we detected specific inflammatory signs. Thus, we observed increased activation of eosinophilic granulocytes. Eosinophilic granulocytes are immune cells that can promote allergies but had not been implicated in common food allergies. The involvement of eosinophils was confirmed by analysis of duodenal fluid that was obtained via a tiny catheter before and after challenge. This showed an increase of a central eosinophil inflammatory mediator: the eosinophilic cationic protein, a product of activated eosinophilic granulocytes. These data indicate that eosinophils are activated in the atypical food allergies, quite in contrast to IgE producing B lymphocytes and IgE binding mast cells in classical allergies. Therefore, atypical food allergies are not only clinically but also mechanistically very different from classical allergies and constitute a separate disease entity.

All patients subsequently received an in-depth dietary consult to avoid those foods that they reacted to. In our first study, patients were followed for 1 year after the endoscopic provocation. Patients filled in validated complaint questionnaires after 3, 6, and 12 months. In the beginning, they had a mean value between 8 and 9 (on a Likert scale from 0 = no complaints to 10 = maximum complaints) that quickly fell to values between 2 and 3 up to the end of the follow-up. Notably, a score of 2–3 is the value of the normal healthy population. The clear identification of the food allergen allowed all study patients to eat normally, except for having to exclude the identified allergen.

To date, our first study is the longest known targeted intervention study in patients with IBS. Previous studies, including studies to test IBS-drugs, usually only lasted for 4–12 weeks. These IBS drugs show some effect in patients with diarrhea- or constipation-predominant IBS but are not dramatically more effective than placebo. Compared to these drugs, the avoidance of the now identified allergens is much more effective. The tested Big Four—wheat, milk, soy, and yeast—are constituents of most foods, especially refined foods. This explains why it has been so difficult to uncover their allergenic potential prior to our method of a challenge with endo-microscopy. Our special diagnostic procedure is not generally available. In practice, we can also do without this complicated procedure in most cases. Patients who improve on the hypoallergenic diet, consisting of potatoes and/or rice, olive oil and salt for 3–5 days, reintroduce pure foods, starting with one of the Big Four, every 2–3 days. If patients develop symptoms with the reintroduction of a certain food, the allergen will be identified. This is a procedure that requires some compliance, which is negligible compared to the untargeted approaches that doctors often recommend or that patients try for themselves, usually with little success. At the same time, we are also working on an easy-to-perform blood test that may allow a diagnostic workup within 1–2 days.

7.5   Summary

Most patients with the diagnosis of IBS are not aware that a food allergy is the cause of their symptoms. Since these symptoms are mainly limited to the GI tract and since classical inflammatory diseases have been excluded, their physicians diagnose IBS. Therapies are still based on untargeted diets, a recommendation for lifestyle changes and stress reduction, or expensive medications. All of these are only modestly effective. We have found that at least 70% of the so-called IBS patients have an underlying definable atypical food allergy. Exclusion of the allergen, mainly wheat, from their diet eliminates their symptoms, a therapeutic success that has never been achieved by any other measure. With approximately 15% of IBS patients in the general population, allergen identification and exclusion will have a smashing effect on healthcare costs and patients' wellbeing.

7.6   Case Vignettes: Wheat Allergies

7.6.1   Patient Mary B. (26 Years): A Special Case of Wheat Allergy

Mary B. (26 years) has been going to the gym regularly for half a year. Four months ago, she noticed increasing shortness of breath with a scratchy feeling in her throat during her training on the running belt. These problems have occurred repeatedly and forced her to stop her training several times prematurely. The symptoms always subside after a few hours of rest at home. She initially attributed the symptoms to a cold, but the problems persisted in the following weeks. Very recently, her shortness of breath was so severe that the staff of the fitness center called an emergency physician who gave her medications that are used for an asthma crisis or an anaphylactic shock. She was admitted as inpatient for 2 days. The standards labs and the cardiovascular status were inconspicuous. She was referred to an allergy specialist for further workup. The usual IgE blood tests for respiratory allergens (pollen, house dust mite, etc.) were all normal. However, such respiratory reactions can also be triggered by drugs such as aspirin or, in rare cases, food, which is why colleagues from allergology contact us. We take a thorough history and Mary tells us that she had not taken any drug that could have caused these problems. However, she states that she usually eats a cheese sandwich 1–2 h before her fitness training. She informs us that usually she has no problems with any kind of food, including cheese and white bread. On the first view, no one would make a connection between the wheat sandwich and her severe respiratory symptoms during exercise. However, there are literature reports of patients that may show a severe allergic reaction to wheat protein only when this is combined with strenuous physical exercise. This allergy does not occur when the same patients consume wheat products while resting. With a possible diagnosis of "wheat-dependent exercise-induced anaphylaxis" (FDEIA), we test Mary's blood for the presence of IgE antibodies to wheat protein, in her case, specifically the omega-gliadins. This test does indeed turn out positive. Because of the severity of her reaction, we recommend Mary to avoid wheat and wheat products altogether. In the follow-up, Mary remains symptom-free and the acute and sometimes life-threatening asthma attacks no longer occur.

Comment on Mary B.

The case of Mary B. (26 years) is a rare form of wheat allergy. Much more common than this form is the so-called baker's asthma that is caused by inhaled flour dust. Baker's asthma affects 8–10% of all bakers who are working in their profession for at least 2 years. Many bakers have to give up their job for this reason; others try to manage their symptoms with anti-allergic drugs and corticosteroids. Acute allergic reactions to wheat consumption are rarer than the inhalative baker's asthma. Both are usually IgE antibody positive. However, the atypical, IgE negative wheat allergy with delayed gastrointestinal symptoms is very frequent, affecting about 4% of the population. Mary has none of these other wheat allergies, but a rare form that only manifests when patients do strenuous exercise shortly before or shortly after they eat wheat products. Her rare form of wheat-dependent exercise-induced anaphylaxis (WDEIA) is due to the fact that the permeability of the intestinal mucosa is briefly increased during strenuous exercise, allowing more potential allergens, in this case wheat, to enter the mucosa and to overcome the usually active tolerance inducing an immune response. The result is a strong mast cell activation, not only in the intestine but also in the lungs, with contraction of the smooth muscles in the airways and severe shortness of breath or asthma. After a few hours of rest, the permeability returns to normal, and the allergic reaction subsides. This condition can become life-threatening, and patients can even die from anaphylactic shock. In general, we have seen that an allergic reaction to usually tolerated foods can arise in otherwise non-allergic people. However, a severe anaphylactic reaction, as in WDEIA, is scarce. To date, it is unclear why this severe reaction is mainly induced by wheat. We hypothesize that the allergy promoting effect of the wheat ATI also promotes this severe reaction to a spectrum to wheat allergens, including omega-gliadins. In this vein, we have shown nutritional ATI fuel nutritional as well as inhalative allergies in general. Now that her diagnosis is clear, Mary can take the appropriate measure by avoiding any wheat consumption shortly before or after her exercise. To be on the safe side, since she had experienced severe anaphylactic episodes, we recommend her to abstain from wheat products completely.

7.6.2   Patient Samuel R. (52 Years): Classic Allergy and Cross-Reaction

Samuel R. (52 years) felt a very unpleasant itching and burning of his palate and tongue, with watering eyes after a working lunch at a conference. Shortly afterward, he experienced increasing shortness of breath. The symptoms were so severe that he had to retire to his hotel room and lie down. He took an anti-allergic which he always carries with him for his wheat allergy that is induced by wheat dust in the air, for example when he enters some bakeries, and—to a lesser extent—after consumption of wheat products that he strictly avoids. He is familiar with the allergy symptoms caused by wheat, namely watering eyes, runny nose and itching and burning of the exposed mucous membranes, usually in combination with asthma. However, he had never experienced such a severe reaction as the critical one described above. In the next 2 h, after having left the conference lunch, he was several times about to call an emergency doctor to his hotel room. Finally, the shortness of breath and the painful burning and itching improved. After another 2 h, the symptoms had completely disappeared, but he started to develop abdominal pain and diarrhea. Samuel reflected on what could have been the cause and is sure that he had not eaten any wheat product, nor been exposed to wheat flour dust. He analyzed what he had eaten before since he is convinced that this must have been a reaction to food. As an appetizer, he had arugula salad with parmesan shavings, lemon and olive oil. The main course was steamed sole fillet in white wine sauce with boiled potatoes and steamed vegetables, followed by a dessert of fruit salad. Immediately, his main suspicion was the fruit salad, since he enjoys salad and fish that he considers healthy and tolerates well. He also knows that heated foods are usually hardly allergenic. The fruit salad, however, contained apple and peach, and he recalled that he always felt slightly inconvenient with these fruits that sometimes cause mild scratching and itching of his oral mucosa, and therefore he avoided to consume the unprocessed fruit. In this case, he was careless and ignored the apple and peach in the other fruits. We know Samuel from 5 years ago when we diagnosed his wheat allergy. After the described life-threatening incident, he presents again in our outpatient clinic. We can indeed confirm IgE antibody positivity to apple and peach, two fruits hat have several common allergens and that also cross-react with some wheat allergens. Cross-reactivity can occur when different allergens have a highly similar structure so that the immune system and the IgE response cannot differentiate between them. From now on, Samuel strictly avoids both fruits in addition to wheat, as he has done intuitively, but not strictly enough before.

Comment on Samuel R.

Samuel R. (52 years) has a classic food allergy with an immediate reaction that results in severe irritation of all mucous membranes. The mucous membranes are the boundaries between the environment and the body. They line the upper and lower digestive tract as well as the inner nose, eyes, palate, throat, and bronchi, those sites that are prominently affected in acute allergies. The most threatening complications of an immediate allergic reaction are severe airway spasm and pharyngeal swelling with shortness of breath up to suffocation. Apart from these severe respiratory symptoms that are mediated by the mucous membranes, another dreaded complication is anaphylactic shock. It results from a sudden and dramatic dilation of blood vessels, induced by histamine and other mediators, leading to severe circulatory complications of life-supporting organs, including the brain and the heart, up to a cardiac arrest. Samuel knows about these complications. Since his symptoms continually worsened, his first idea was to call the emergency team. Indeed, that would have been the right measure. Instead, he took his anti-allergic medication, and it was only good luck that with this relatively weak intervention, his condition stabilized and finally improved. Patients with severe allergies always carry with them an emergency kit, such as an epi-pen, i.e., an easy-to-apply injection of adrenaline or epinephrine, hormones that on the one hand relax the ring muscles of the respiratory tract, and on the other hand contract the dilated blood vessels. If applied early enough, this injection can prevent excessive swelling of the mucosal membranes and bronchial vasoconstriction and thereby facilitate respiration. It can also prevent the development of anaphylactic shock. In addition to the epi-pen, it is also recommended to take a high single dose of corticosteroids that downregulate the excessive inflammatory response of the mucosal membranes in severe allergic reactions.

The question arises, why Samuel, who has a proven wheat allergy, has developed an allergic reaction to apple and peach. It is frequently observed that allergic patients develop allergy another on top of the primary one. The reason for this phenomenon is the so-called cross-reactivity of specific allergens that derive from different foods. Some allergens of wheat have a similar structure as the main allergens of apple and peach. Therefore, the IgE antibodies produced against wheat (by B lymphocytes) do not only bind to the wheat allergens but also to the similar apple and peach allergens. The binding affinity of the wheat IgE to the cross-reactive apple and peach allergens can increase over time. In Samuel's case, this explains the gradual increase of his allergic reaction to the apple and peach allergens. The major cross-reactive allergens in wheat, apple and peach are so-called lipid transfer proteins that play a role in the fat metabolism of plants.

In general, the occurrence and spontaneous disappearance of allergies, especially food allergies, is very complicated and still incompletely understood. We assume that allergy patients who strictly avoid certain foods develop a particularly strong reaction to the allergenic and cross-reactive foods, while patients with a less strict allergen avoidance can develop a certain degree of tolerance. This is also how the principle of oral hypo-sensitization works that is medically used to induce tolerance in allergic patients. Other methods of hypo-sensitization use subcutaneous injection of small doses of the allergen, such as pollen, animal hair or insect allergens. Tolerization by hypo-sensitization may take several years of regular allergen application to be effective. However, it is strongly advised not to experiment with oral or other hypo-sensitizations without the help of an expert, since, as the case of Samuel shows, uncontrollable and life-threatening reactions can occur. Samuel's case and the tricky balance between tolerance and an excessive immune response illustrate the complexity of immune regulation in the mucosal membranes.

7.6.3   Sylvia H. (48 Years): From Irritable Bowel Syndrome to Atypical Food Allergy

Sylvia H. (48 years) had repetitive episodes of abdominal pain, sometimes combined with diarrhea or severe constipation, for the last 5 years. She also complained about general discomfort and nausea. Sylvia is a business school graduate and works as a tax consultant on a freelance basis. She describes her work as fulfilling and enjoyable. Her marriage is harmonious, as is her relationship with her daughter, who has already left home for college. Sylvia's history does not reveal any prior severe illnesses. Due to her persistent abdominal symptoms, her internist had ordered a large number of tests, including the antibody test for celiac disease, stool tests for viral or bacterial infectious diseases, for parasites and chronic inflammatory bowel disease (stool calprotectin), and breath tests for fructose and lactose intolerance. Moreover, an upper and lower endoscopy, as well as an abdominal computerized tomography (CT), were performed. All these tests and examinations yielded normal results, as did a subsequent broad screening for food allergies via skin scratch tests and blood tests for IgE antibodies. Based on this battery of negative tests and examinations, Sylvia had received the diagnose of irritable bowel syndrome (IBS), a diagnostic label that is commonly given to all patients with abdominal complaints but negative test results. As the treatment of choice, her internist advised her to avoid coffee and hot spices, to follow a balanced diet with regular meals, and to reduce excessive stress. Sylvia followed these instructions and changed her lifestyle. However, her abdominal symptoms did not improve. After 6 weeks of frustrating attempts to optimally adhere to the recommendations and dietary advice, without symptom improvement, she presents in our outpatient clinic. She has read about novel allergy tests and asks us if it would make sense to have done an IgG test for food allergens, a test that would not be covered by her health insurance. We strongly advise against this test, as it usually produces false-positive as well as false-negative results. Reviewing her medical records, we can confirm that inflammatory bowel diseases, as well as celiac disease, can be ruled out. We perform a thorough physical examination and take a detailed history that is inconspicuous, except for a bloated abdomen and mild pain in the upper abdomen on deep palpation. We also ask for previous abdominal surgery and journeys to subtropical or tropical regions. Sylvia reports that 6 years ago, shortly before the onset of her symptoms, she went on a three-week trip to Mexico. We arrange for a glucose hydrogen breath test that is useful to diagnose abnormal bacterial colonization of the small intestine since some patients develop a persistent small intestinal dysbiosis (colonization with pathogenic bacteria) after a stay in the tropics or subtropics. This "small intestinal bacterial overgrowth" (SIBO) causes nausea and abdominal pain, often combined with diarrhea. SIBO can also occur after an abdominal surgery that may result in impaired intestinal motility, which favors dysbiosis. SIBO can usually be treated with certain antibiotics over extended periods. Sylvia's glucose breath test is negative, and therefore, SIBO can be ruled out. Her history also reveals that she follows a fasting diet every year in spring, living only from vegetable broths, juices and teas for 2 weeks.

During this diet, she always feels much better and essentially pain-free. In everyday life, however, the problems return, and pain and bloating are prominent 30 min to 1 h after breakfast, much to her disappointment, since she has designed a particularly healthy breakfast consisting of a freshly prepared 5-grain-muesli, fresh fruits, organic milk, and natural yogurt. At noon, she regularly feels fatigued and is hardly able to work. We suspect that she may have an IgE antibody negative, i.e., an atypical food allergy. We include her in one of our studies of IBS/food sensitive patients. This study applies the special endoscopic technique of confocal laser endo-microscopy. We apply the four most prevalent allergens in temporal sequence to the small intestinal mucosa, followed by 5 min of observation after each application. What we observe, is an immediate inflammatory reaction after application of a wheat suspension, while the other tested foods, milk, soy, and yeast, do not trigger an inflammatory response. This confirms the diagnosis of an atypical wheat allergy. Sylvia receives a dietary consult that informs her how to carry out a wheat-free diet. Already after 2 weeks of the diet that she had to extend also to other gluten-containing cereals, Sylvia's symptoms have almost resolved. After another year, we see her again, and she has remained symptom-free on the wheat- and gluten-free diet.

Comment on Sylvia H.

Sylvia H. (48 years) has a long history of abdominal complaints. Since extensive texts and examinations did not yield pathological results, she was diagnosed with IBS. As in many patients with this diagnosis, standard dietary and lifestyle-advise did not lead to improvement of her symptoms. When we see her, we first rule out "small intestinal bacterial overgrowth" (SIBO), a frequently missed diagnosis in patients who have traveled to the tropics or the subtropics or who have a small intestinal motility problem, e.g., after an abdominal operation. This test was negative. Notably, she reported that she was feeling much better when she pursued her spring fasting diet. We, therefore, suspected that she had a delayed, IgE antibody negative, i.e., atypical food allergy.

There is no simple test to indicate the presence of an atypical allergy. IgE antibody and skin tests are negative. The commercially available IgG tests are useless and misleading since positive test results usually indicate tolerance instead of an allergy. Our patient has the unique possibility to participate in our study, employing the technology of confocal endo-microscopy after the food challenge. We apply suspensions/emulsions of four common foods (wheat, milk, soy, and yeast) to the small intestinal mucosa. These four foods are responsible for two-thirds of the atypical allergies. Sylvia's healthy breakfast contained at least two of these allergens, namely wheat and milk. Notably, wheat and milk are the first and second most frequent atypical allergens, respectively. Indeed, we can positively prove that Sylvia is allergic to wheat.

Symptoms of an atypical food allergy improve on fasting or on a hypoallergenic diet, such as potatoes or rice combined with olive oil and salt, a diet that we prescribe to patients, in order to confirm an atypical allergy. This diet is easy to follow for 3–5 days. If symptoms improve, an atypical food allergy is likely. Since we usually cannot perform the complex endoscopic method of small intestinal allergen challenge, combined with confocal laser endo-microscopy to directly demonstrate the reaction to a specific food, we rather instruct our patients to reintroduce defined and pure foods every 2–3 days. This way we can identify the food allergens, starting with the most frequent one, wheat, within a few days up to a few weeks.

Although the patient must follow a diet similar to that of celiac disease, i.e., avoidance of gluten-containing foods, the mechanisms are different. While in celiac disease only gluten proteins trigger an inflammatory T lymphocyte reaction in the intestine, wheat allergies are caused by many different proteins, including gluten and other protein classes, such as wheat albumins and globulins that stimulate IgE production in classical allergies or eosinophil activation in atypical allergies.

7.6.4   Summary of the Cases with Wheat Allergies

We describe three cases of allergic reactions to food. The first is a rare case of a classical wheat allergy, namely, "wheat-dependent exercise-induced anaphylaxis" (WDEIA). This case illustrates that the susceptibility to food allergies increases, at least temporarily, during strenuous physical exercise. The second case demonstrates that in classical food allergies, an expansion of the allergic response to other foods can develop when the allergens show structural similarity (cross-reactivity). This can lead to life-threatening complications, even if the primary allergen is strictly avoided. The third case is a good example of a typical ordeal of patients with an atypical food allergy. These patients undergo numerous and repetitive tests and endoscopies that yield negative results. They then receive the final diagnosis of IBS. Dietary and lifestyle changes to treat IBS are usually of little or no benefit. Current drugs that address diarrhea- or constipation-predominant IBS can help but are only slightly superior to placebo treatments. In our clinical studies, we have found that 70% of IBS patients have an atypical food allergy that can be positively demonstrated by the technique of confocal laser endo-microscopy. In clinical practice, patients who improve on a hypo-allergenic diet can reintroduce every 2–3 days to identify their allergen. Exclusion of the detected allergen is the most effective therapy for these patients who incorrectly received the diagnosis of IBS, but in fact have an atypical food allergy.

Chapter 8
It's Not Always Wheat!

In the preceding chapters, we have demonstrated that wheat, gluten, and ATI are responsible for a large number of diagnoses and diseases. However, we do not want to leave the impression that wheat-sensitivities are the only culprit of all ailments, as many non-scientific bestselling books suggest. It is not acceptable to use a "one-fits-all diagnosis" and give consequential therapeutic recommendations that incriminate wheat as the sole and central villain. The underlying unscientific mindset will do more harm than good. The complexity of most diseases requires a thorough and broad understanding of the human body, the immune system, and medicine in general.

As the cases in this chapter will show, a thorough diagnostic workup is mandatory to understand and appropriately treat complex diseases that require broad medical knowledge and clinical experience. Only with this body of knowledge, it is possible to consider the important differential diagnoses. Any attempt to shorten the laborious and time-consuming diagnostic path, which has to include an in-depth history taking and a hand-on physical examination, comes close to professional malpractice. Thus, we frequently see patients who have fallen victim to this simplified diagnostic and therapeutic path, since they do not have a wheat-induced disease, despite some typical symptoms of wheat-sensitivity. For these patients, staying on a wheat-free diet may lead to some improvement, but also to omission of necessary further diagnostic and therapeutic measures that would address the major underlying though undetected disease.

© Springer Nature Switzerland AG 2019
D. Schuppan, K. Gisbert-Schuppan, *Wheat Syndromes*
https://doi.org/10.1007/978-3-030-19023-1_8

8.1 Case Vignettes: Patients with Diseases that Superficially Look Like Wheat-Sensitivity

8.1.1 Patient Curt W. (20 Years): Incorrect Diagnosis of Celiac Disease in Childhood

Curt W. (20 years), a physics undergraduate, had been diagnosed with celiac disease at the age of 6 when he developed severe abdominal pain and diarrhea over several weeks. Due to the protracted abdominal symptoms, his pediatrician had an endoscopy performed. The pediatrician had informed Curt's parents that the biopsy finding of the endoscopy indicated celiac disease. The parents received a consult on how to manage the gluten-free diet. Since Curt's symptoms improved within 2 weeks of the diet, the diagnosis seemed to be confirmed. The entire family adapted to a gluten-free household. His parents have always been very conscientious about this diet. They have taken care that Curt was protected from any contact with gluten, i.e., he was not allowed to eat out or with other families or to freely enjoy company or birthday parties when ice cream, cake or cookies were offered. Instead, he always had to bring along his own rice crackers, and he always felt marginalized. For many years, he never questioned these regulations. However, since he had left home for college, the young patient repeatedly permitted himself—with a spirit of rebellion as he concedes—dietary transgressions, as he tells us. Especially when he joins his friends in eating a piece of pizza or a cookie. He also does not pay attention anymore whether prepared foods may contain some gluten, including lunch at the cafeteria. He is positively surprised that he has not developed any symptoms. Therefore, he has begun to question the diagnosis of celiac disease and visits our clinic, asking us of a re-evaluation of his celiac diagnosis. When we see him, we find out that the report of his endoscopy and biopsy at age six is not available anymore. We also do not know if the endomysium antibodies (EMA) or the celiac disease-specific antibodies to transglutaminase—this test just became available at that time—were determined. We, therefore, arrange for basic blood work, including the transglutaminase auto-antibodies and a blood test for the genetic predisposition: HLA-DQ2 or HLD-DQ8. The standard laboratory tests are normal, but he is a carrier of HLA-DQ2, the major genetic predisposition for celiac disease. However, this does not prove that Curt has celiac disease indeed. The possibility remains that his abdominal crisis at age 6 might not have been due to celiac disease, but rather to a prolonged bacterial or viral enteritis that would have improved spontaneously. We, therefore, suggest that he now eats a normal, gluten-containing diet for at least 4 weeks. This means he should eat at least 2–3 slices of bread or a comparable amount of other gluten-containing foods per day. Should significant complaints arise before the end of the 4-week-provocation, Curt is instructed to stop the gluten-challenge and inform us. After 4 weeks, we see Curt again. He reports that he does not feel any discomfort on the gluten-containing diet. His transglutaminase antibodies are still in the normal range, and upper endoscopy and biopsies show no evidence of inflammation or villus atrophy. This makes celiac disease highly unlikely and allows him to continue the normal, gluten-containing diet. We see him again after 1 year. All laboratory tests, including the transglutaminase antibodies, continue to be normal. This confirms with great certainty that Curt does indeed not have celiac disease. Curt and his family had been living with the misdiagnosis of celiac disease for almost 15 years.

Commentary on Curt W.
Curt W. (20 years) had a protracted intestinal infection as a child. These infections usually heal after a few days up to 2 weeks. Rarely, however, they can last longer and also show the histological picture of celiac disease. In case of viral or bacterial enteritis, EMA or transglutaminase antibodies are negative or only marginally elevated. Obviously, these antibodies have not been determined when the supposed celiac disease was diagnosed. After the negative gluten challenge of 4 weeks and its extension to 1 year, we can clearly rule out celiac disease, although the patient is a carrier of the genetic predisposition HLA-DQ2. In Curt's history, we can see how far-reaching and formative an incorrect diagnosis can become in a sensitive period of life.

8.1.2 Patient Nicole R. (47 Years): Inborn Immune Deficiency

Nicole R. (47 years) is an administrative employee and mother of two grown-up daughters. She comes to our office after referral by another tertiary care center together with her husband and a big stack of medical records. In early adolescence, she had been diagnosed with common variable immunodeficiency (CVID), i.e., her immune cells produce insufficient amounts of immunoglobulins. In her wording, she "continuously" has flulike symptoms, often also more severe respiratory infections, even during the warmer seasons of the year. To support her immune system, her primary care physician gives her regular injections of immunoglobulin every 4 weeks. For 2 years now, she increasingly has periods of diarrhea, and her labs show a vitamin and protein deficiency. Moreover, she is severely fatigued, to such a degree that she "could immediately go to bed again after breakfast".

She considers herself physically and psychologically frail and experiences her professional as well as her private life as compromised. The already slim patient has lost 22 lb (10 kg) in 3 months and her current BMI of 18 places her in the underweight range. Her gastroenterologist acted appropriately when he performed an upper endoscopy 2 years ago. He found a highly active celiac disease with histological Marsh class IIIc, indicating severe inflammatory damage. The transglutaminase antibodies were only mildly elevated. From then on, she started a strictly gluten-free diet and completely rearranged her household. However, neither her condition nor her physical fitness improved with these measures. Thus, diarrhea and her continuous weight loss did not subside. For further workup, her gastroenterologist referred her to the tertiary care center nearby. Another upper endoscopy was performed that again yielded severe celiac disease of stage Marsh IIIc. The patient and her attending physicians turn to us for expert advice. When we see the patient, we first explain to her that it is crucial to confirm or rule out refractory celiac disease, a severe condition that sometimes can only be treated with immunosuppressive medication. We perform another upper endoscopy, this time reaching further down into small intestine with multiple biopsies for specialized histological, immunological and molecular analyses. Moreover, a computerized tomography (CT) of the abdomen is ordered. We can exclude a refractory coeliac disease since there are no further diagnostic clues in the endoscopically accessible sections of the small intestine. Equally, the abdominal CT does not show a tumorous lesion or enlarged lymph nodes. We then check if the patient is a carrier of the genetic celiac predisposition. Unexpectedly, she is negative for HLA-DQ2 and HLA-DQ8, excluding celiac disease. Therefore, we consider differential diagnoses. As we already know, she has an immunodeficiency, i.e., a genetic deficiency in immunoglobulins. Notably, her blood levels of the major immunoglobulin IgG have been in the lower range of 20–40% of the average normal IgG levels, despite regular substitution. This usually secures sufficient protection for patients with CVID. There are, however, rare cases of patients with this genetic disease who develop marked villous atrophy that is difficult to distinguish from celiac disease. The underlying mechanisms are not entirely clear but may relate to a disturbed intestinal immune regulation towards intestinal microbes and nutrients. Our recommendation is to increase the substitution of immunoglobulin G. In her case, applying the dose in every 2 instead of every 4 weeks in the hope that this would allow her intestine to heal. After 3 weeks, we see her again. Her appearance has changed amazingly. She tells us that only 2 days after the extra dose of IgG diarrhea had stopped and since then her bowel movements have normalized. Equally, her fatigue is gone, and her original vigor and optimism have returned. She has also gained 4.4 lb (2 kg) in weight. Moreover, the has the feeling that her flulike symptoms have disappeared and, as she says, "I can breathe freely for the first time in years".

Comment on Nicole R.

Nicole R. (47 years) has a rare genetic disorder of the immune system, common variable immunodeficiency (CVID). Her plasma cells produce insufficient amounts of immunoglobulins that are important for the defense against pathogens, but also the regulation of the immune system in the gut. Infections or complication in these patients can usually be prevented by infusions or injections of immunoglobulin G every few weeks to achieve blood levels between 20 and 50% of normal. It is unclear why some of these patients develop small intestinal inflammation resembling celiac disease. We hypothesize that these patients are either more sensitive to microbial pathogens that infect the gut or develop an autoimmune process in the small intestinal mucosa that is favored by low immunoglobulin levels. There are reports that immunoglobulin substitution can dampen autoimmune diseases. In this sense, our strategy to further increase Nicole's immunoglobulin level was successful. In her case, the gluten-free diet does not improve the situation. Equally, ATI rather play a minor role in this kind of inflammation.

8.1.3   *Patient Emily D. (70 Years): Severe Small Intestinal Damage Due to a Medication*

Emily D. (70 years) is a recently widowed, retired high-school director, who is referred to us with the diagnosis of refractory celiac disease by a gastroenterologist in private practice. When we see her the first time, she is accompanied by her daughter. Emily reports that she has been living with the diagnosis of celiac disease when she retired, a transition in her life that is still difficult to cope with for her. With this life event, she developed diarrhea and abdominal cramps. Since the diagnosis of celiac disease, she adheres to a strict gluten-free diet. However, the diet has had little effect, and her diarrhea and abdominal pain persist. Her general practitioner first attributes her complaints to the patient's critical life events, e.g., the loss of her husband 2 years ago in combination with her retirement, and suspects an underlying psychosomatic dynamic. However, Emily does not accept this interpretation, although she still experiences her loss as extremely painful and mourns persistently. She refuses the antidepressant that her doctor had suggested to her. The last upper endoscopy a week ago showed a pronounced celiac disease, histologically Marsh IIIb. Emily asserts that she strictly follows the gluten-free diet and "never" deviated from it, which is no longer difficult for her. Her labs reveal decreased levels of vitamin B12, vitamin D and folic acid and a substantial iron deficiency anemia. Furthermore, she is a carrier of HLA-DQ2, the genetic predisposition of celiac disease. These labs are all well compatible with severe celiac disease. Accordingly, Emily complains of continuous tiredness and fatigue. She is also apprehensive about a recent finding of severe osteoporosis (T-value = −4; a value of −2 already indicates osteoporosis). Osteoporosis is also a typical complication of untreated celiac disease. Based on these data, we perform several examinations: another upper endoscopy with multiple biopsy sampling for special analyses, an imaging of the small intestine (MR enterography), and an a computerized abdominal tomography (CT). These examinations permit an evaluation of those parts of the small intestine that cannot be reached with the upper endoscope. Besides, the CT allows an assessment of the lymph nodes that surround the intestine. In refractory celiac disease type 2 and especially in its advanced form, intestinal T cell lymphoma, marked inflammation and ulceration in the lower small intestine, as well as enlarged abdominal lymph nodes, are found. Fortunately for Emily, these imaging studies were unremarkable, ruling out refractory celiac disease or lymphoma.

On closer inspection of the many medications that Emily has been taking for years, including drugs for mild type 2 diabetes and hypertension, one medication catches our attention. It is Olmesartan, an anti-hypertensive drug belonging to the class of angiotensin receptor blockers. Notably, Olmesartan has recently been associated with small intestinal damage and symptoms resembling celiac disease. We discontinue Olmesartan, replace it with another anti-hypertensive, and substitute vitamins and iron. With these measures, Emily's complaints rapidly improve. After 3 months, she is completely symptom-free, and a control endoscopy shows a near normalization of her small intestinal mucosa. In exchange with us, she carefully resumes a normal, gluten-containing diet. This dietary change does not cause any diarrhea or other symptoms. After 1 year, we see her again. She has no complaints on the normal, gluten-containing diet and feels healthy and energetic. The control endoscopy shows complete regeneration of the small intestine. She has won back her energy and optimism and regained her life balance, including community work, where she is engaged in afternoon tutoring and homework support for children.

Commentary on Emily D.

Emily D. (70 years) had been diagnosed with celiac disease, but her complaints did not improve on a strict gluten-free diet. Therefore, she was referred to us for suspected refractory celiac disease, a possible diagnosis when the patient does not improve on the gluten-free diet. With additional testing and procedures, we can exclude refractory celiac disease type 2 or its advanced stage intestinal T cell lymphoma. We are happy about these results, since these complications are usually associated with a bad prognosis, in case of T cell lymphoma of only up to a few years with conventional chemotherapy. Taking Emily's history, we discover that her antihypertensive medication, Olmesartan, is the cause of her intestinal inflammation with villous atrophy and treatment-resistant diarrhea, malabsorption, and abdominal pain. Olmesartan was only recently reported to cause such problems in some patients; problems that are indistinguishable from celiac disease at first glance. The underlying mechanism is largely unclear, but one study showed that this class of drugs might act via inhibition of transforming growth factor β (TGF-β1), a central immunosuppressive cytokine.

After discontinuation of Olmesartan, small intestinal inflammation subsides, and the clinical symptoms disappear. Still, celiac disease cannot be ruled out completely in this case because Emily is a carrier of HLA-DQ2, a central genetic predisposition. She carefully resumes a normal, gluten-containing diet which indeed does not cause any problems. Moreover, the labs and endoscopic control after 1 year remain inconspicuous. Therefore, we can conclude that Emily does not have celiac disease and the antihypertensive drug Olmesartan caused her complaints and clinical picture.

8.1.4 Patient David P. (39 Years): Chronic Inflammatory Bowel Disease

David P. (39 years) sees us for a special consultation. He is already in treatment with a gastroenterologist in private practice for several years. He works as a police officer, mainly on patrol. He was diagnosed with ulcerative colitis at age 20. Currently, he has increasing problems on patrol due to an exacerbation of his colitis that goes along with uncontrollable, partly bloody diarrhea. After the first disease manifestation 19 years ago that was treated with high doses of corticosteroids, his colitis remained in remission for many years, with low disease activity, occasional mild diarrhea, and abdominal pain. With a so-called maintenance therapy with the oral drug 5-ASA, his colitis was well-controlled, except for another exacerbation at age 30 that could also be controlled with a high dose of corticosteroids for several weeks. 3 months ago, his ulcerative colitis worsened again. Since then, David has diarrhea up to 8 times a day, anemia and elevated inflammation markers in blood and stools. In these last 3 months, the slim and physically active police officer loses 6.6 lb (3 kg) of weight. He is not able to go on patrol anymore because of repeated abdominal cramps and diarrhea. Colonoscopy showed a pan-colitis, i.e., inflammation of the whole large intestine. This time, the therapy with high dose corticosteroids was only marginally effective. Therefore, his gastroenterologist began treatment with an antibody against TNF-α (tumor necrosis factor α). TNF-α is a central mediator of inflammation in chronic inflammatory bowel diseases, i.e., ulcerative colitis and Crohn's disease. David presents 6 weeks after the start of the TNF-α therapy, 2 days before this third injection. This therapy is usually given at time points 0, 2, 6, and then every 8 weeks as a single injection over several months or even years. He tells us that his symptoms have only improved modestly since then and that he still has to deal with 3–4 daily episodes of often bloody and painful diarrhea. He asks us if it would make sense to start the ATI-reduced diet, of which he has heard in the media. Based on our studies, we recommend beginning the ATI-reduced diet in support of his ongoing antibody therapy. We see him 2 months later when we give him the fourth dose of the TNF-α-antibody. Unfortunately, his symptoms have not improved. He still experiences diarrhea 3–4 times a day, sometimes bloody, and he feels exhausted. We recommend that he continue with the ATI-reduced diet. When we see him again after another 2 months for his fifth TNF-α treatment, he reports a marked improvement, now with non-bloody, regular bowel movements, a slight weight gain, and a significantly improved performance, allowing him to work on patrol again. We now prescribe the drugs azathioprine and 5-ASA to maintain remission and give him another 2 doses of the TNF-α antibody over the following 4 months. 6 months later, his disease is still in remission. He is so glad about his improvement that he wants to continue the ATI-reduced diet. We explain to him that yet we do not have conclusive clinical data that the ATI-reduced diet will maintain remission on its own. Based on our scientific data, we believe it makes sense to continue the ATI-reduced diet in conjunction with the remission-maintaining drugs. The diet is not difficult to carry out, and David likes his dietary change.

Commentary on David P.

David P. (39 years) has a severe exacerbation of ulcerative colitis, a chronic inflammatory bowel disease that primarily affects the large intestine. He shows the typical symptoms: bloody diarrhea, anemia, impairment of his general wellbeing and ability to work, and weight loss. Colonoscopy demonstrates a pan-colitis, an inflammation of the entire large intestine. He initially received treatment with high doses of corticosteroid that led to remission, i.e., a significant improvement over a longer period. For several years now, so-called biologicals—antibodies against inflammatory factors—have been available for patients. These antibodies often lead to disease remission even in corticosteroid-resistant patients. David has received such therapy with TNF-α antibodies, with little effect at first. Most patients recover after the first or second dose of such a biological. If a patient with ulcerative colitis does not respond to one of these novel therapies, a serious operation is usually discussed: a colectomy, the removal of the entire large intestine. It is therefore understandable that David is looking for further treatment options. He learns from the media that ATI promote inflammatory processes, including inflammatory bowel disease. Although we are just beginning to perform controlled clinical studies, our mechanistic lab data and observations in individual patients suggest that the ATI-reduced diet should benefit David. Initially, the modest clinical improvement after 2 months of the diet, that goes along with the continued TNF-α antibody therapy, is disappointing. Likely, that the severity of the intestinal inflammation is so pronounced that the effect of the ATI-reduced diet is rather small in this acute phase, especially also in combination with the highly effective biological drug. The ATI-reduced diet may rather be effective in the treatment of mild to moderate colitis or the maintenance of remission. Fortunately, the patient's severe colitis was ultimately controlled. Here, the contribution of ATI reduction is difficult to assess in view of the specific anti-inflammatory drug, i.e., the TNF-α antibody. Nonetheless, we can assume that the ATI-reduced diet plays an important role in maintaining remission and improving therapeutic response.[1]

8.1.5   Summary

The unifying theme that underlies the first three cases presented in this chapter is that wheat, gluten, or ATI were believed to have caused disease. Patients were referred to us by specialists. These cases demonstrate that prior to dietary recommendations, a thorough diagnostic workup and assessment is needed. They also illustrate that the astonishing novel findings and successes in food- and especially wheat-related diseases that we present in this book cannot be generalized uncritically, i.e., they are not always the magic bullet that cures all diseases or symptoms.

The case of David demonstrates that the ATI-reduced diet alone cannot be expected to heal severe and acute inflammatory diseases upfront. Rather, acute exacerbations usually require highly effective immune-modulatory drugs. In any case, the ATI-reduced diet should be started in parallel and plays a crucial role in maintaining remission.

This chapter is meant as a reminder that in medicine when it comes to the treatment of the individual patient, there is never a simple recipe. As we point out during the entire course of our book, even with the ground-breaking novel discoveries that we present, an optimal and personalized therapy always requires in-depth knowledge of the diseases and their mechanisms, the complex interactions of the organ systems, and a meticulous follow-up of the disease course.

---

[1] Based on our research, the same obviously applies to other severe inflammatory diseases, such as rheumatoid arthritis, multiple sclerosis, Crohn's disease or lupus, that also require highly effective immunomodulatory drugs during acute exacerbations.

Chapter 9
Outlook

After reading our book, we hope you will agree with us that our findings and the consequences for medicine are deeply transformational. For us, it is clear that we would not have been able to produce our scientific results and to assess their significance for medical practice within a standard healthcare routine. Therefore, we would like to give an outlook that may help medical practitioners to find their way of dealing adequately with the complexity of the human body and human beings in a holistic and integrated manner. The only way that can do justice to the kind of diseases we are dealing with today and on which we have shed light on in this book.

9.1 Clinical Practice

Our clinical work combines a high level of expertise in many disease areas, a broad understanding of the body's immune system, consideration of the important role of environmental factors, such as lifestyle, nutrition, and the intestinal microbiome, as well as an understanding of the biographical and psychosocial aspects of the patient. All these factors constitute an interconnecting system that finally determines the patient's health or disease. Based on our clinical experience from decades, we are sure that an effective and long-term cure, or at least an improvement of many diseases, for which no therapy existed before or whose treatment has been unsatisfactory, is often possible with easy measures, once the disease triggers and their interactions have been defined. With the knowledge and deep understanding of the underlying mechanisms, these diseases can now be classified and effectively treated with strikingly simple measures. In much detail, we have described these novel, usually severe disease entities that are triggered or promoted by the wrong food. We have reported on how they left patients in despair, with ineffective remedies and limited help even by specialist doctors. Moreover, we have shown that their treatment can be managed just by the omission of the identified food trigger. Even in autoimmune diseases, these treatments can be more effective than current and most modern

© Springer Nature Switzerland AG 2019

D. Schuppan, K. Gisbert-Schuppan, *Wheat Syndromes*

https://doi.org/10.1007/978-3-030-19023-1_9

pharmacological therapies. We have organized our outpatient clinic in a novel way, in order to uphold this level of highly patient-oriented and personalized medicine.

What we're doing clinically in practice is first taking painstaking, but not rampant histories, leaving room for the patients to tell us about their feelings and opinions in regard to their disease trajectory. This includes events and coincidences when their disease became apparent or got worse. This aspect of narrative medicine is central to the identification of diseases and disease-promoting factors that otherwise may get out of focus for both, the treating physician and the affected patient. It is equally important for the patient to understand what is going on and be able to make sense of the disease, in order to better cope with it.

We communicate with our patients, before they first present in our outpatient clinic, and make sure that they collect relevant prior medical records, lab results, and reports of clinical procedures. On first encounter with every new patient, we also perform an in-depth physical exam, since—as experience has taught us—prior exams may have been superficial or have missed important signs and findings that are needed for our diagnostic process. If indicated, we order additional blood, urinary or stool tests, and endoscopic or imaging studies that we deem relevant to confirm or reject specific diagnoses, even for rare diseases, that may have escaped prior attention.

All relevant findings, the preliminary diagnosis, a therapeutic plan and measures to be taken, are recorded during the patient's visit, explained in detail, and handed out as a copy to the patient and his or her treating PCP or specialist right at the first visit. This includes handouts for our standardized and evidence-based dietary procedures, like the hypo-allergenic diet with potato/rice, olive oil, and salt and the gradual testing-in of other foods, the ATI-reduced diet, or the strict gluten-free diet in newly discovered celiac disease. Patients are also connected to the relevant self-support organizations, such as the national celiac society or autoimmune networks.

Since our patients usually travel long distances to see us, they and their PCPs or local specialists are asked to have some of the laboratory tests and especially endoscopic and imaging studies done locally, close to their home. We offer them and their local physicians, to stay in contact with us, preferentially via email. We use (password-protected) email to quickly inform the patients about the lab results of their last visit combined with an explanatory note. This includes the medical monitoring of the patients' dietary and pharmacological measures, to optimize therapeutic outcome and modify the diagnostic and therapeutic strategy if indicated. More complex issues are discussed personally on the phone. More rarely, we see patients with a worrisome health condition, a suspected malignancy or an exacerbation of a severe inflammatory disease that require immediate diagnostic work-up, usually with endoscopy and imaging, and a targeted anti-inflammatory or anti-cancer treatment. In these cases, we arrange for immediate inpatient admission.

Overall, our patient care differs from the conventional patterns of outpatient medicine. First, we devote unusually much time to each patient, an average of 1–4 h for each novel case, in order to get at the root of his or her medical problem. Second, we consider a broad range of differential diagnoses, even if they at first glance do not appear to be connected to the major complaints of the patient; here, our considerations always include the patient's perception of the disease and socio-psychological factors. Third, we apply our novel and evidence-based diagnostic and therapeutic dietary measures to the newly unraveled disease entities like ATI-sensitivity and atypical food allergies.

The medicine that we provide is not reimbursed adequately since current reimbursement by healthcare providers is mainly based on blood tests, procedures, and complex pharmacological therapies. In contrast, the expert clinic that we practice does not lead to high material or procedural costs. However, it is highly effective for both, the patients who can be cured of long-term and highly compromising illness, and the healthcare providers that will save huge costs. These healthcare costs are incurred by repetitive and unnecessary tests and procedures, on top of frequent ineffective and unnecessary pharmacological therapies, not to speak of the unwanted side-effects. Compared to many drug treatments, we practice affordable medicine with high efficacy. Here, the time and expertise that we invest in our patients do by far outperform conventional measures, when it comes to both, the patients' benefit and the costs for society and the healthcare system. Dissemination of this knowledge to patients, doctors and policymakers, and prospective "cost-benefit" calculations are an important task that should lead to adequate reimbursement for informed and dedicated physicians.

We are aware that we work against the trend of time that favors over-specialization and generates physicians who "know all about nothing", but not much about the complexity of human beings and the complexity of diseases. Our doctor for the future is both specialist and generalist. In the field covered here the specialization is gastroenterology that traditionally and originally was tightly linked to endocrinology and immunology. Both are disciplines that require a detailed and updated knowledge about the cellular and immunological processes that take place in the gut and that affect the rest of the body. This includes autoimmune diseases that for a long time have been seen as autonomous and genetically determined immune derangements that require a brute force of pharmacological immune suppression. Our doctor for the future should be aware and take active notice that autoimmune processes are centrally influenced and modulated by specific nutritional factors and the intestinal microbes.

Our book is supposed to be an encouragement and a groundbreaking step in the direction of what we think medicine is supposed to be like. In describing our clinical practice, we would like to encourage doctors and other responsible persons in the healthcare system to seize, enable, and promote conceptions like ours. We can assure healthcare professionals that it is deeply satisfying and delightful to work with such a comprehensive and profound practical approach.

9.2 Aspects of Further Research

Another important activity that we pursue is the assessment of the pathogenic potential of cereals that are consumed worldwide, especially wheat. In 4 ongoing collaborative research projects, funded by the government and the food industry, we investigate the ATI content, their inflammatory activity, and the allergenic potential of several hundred variants of wheat and relative grains. These results are just emerging and still unpublished; but we can already state that ATI activity can vary markedly, severalfold, between different wheat species, despite similar yield and quality. This is quite different from gluten whose content and immunogenic properties in celiac disease, remain fairly constant. Moreover, ATI activity is affected by the site and time of cultivation. With this information, we will soon be able to select wheat variants with low ATI activity and disease-promoting potential. In addition, further ATI-reduction is possible with extractive methods and specific breeding, possibly bringing the ATI down to less than 10% of a standard wheat product, the arbitrary threshold that we have set for our patients. Importantly, the gluten would be left untouched, since it is not harmful to patients with ATI-sensitivity, and since it is important for the good taste and texture of bakery products.

However, as long as we have to deal with normal and uncontrolled cereals, we hope to raise awareness for the affected patients and promote a better understanding of their symptoms that need to be taken seriously and diagnosed as what they are: wheat syndromes that can be improved or even cured by simple dietary measures. Table 9.1 highlights major clinical features that allow to differentiate the wheat sensitivities.

Table 9.1 Differences between the wheat sensitivities and FODMAP intolerance

	Celiac Disease	ATI-Sensitivity	Atypical Wheat Allergy	FODMAP-Intolerance
Time interval from wheat exposure to onset of symptoms	Days-weeks	Hours-days	Minutes-hours	Minutes-hours
Pathogenesis	T cell immunity to gluten	Innate Immunity to ATI	**Many proteins →** T-cells, Mast cells, Eosinophils	**Many** (complex) **carbohydrates**
HLA	HLA DQ2/8 restricted	Not HLA DQ2/8 restricted	Not HLA DQ2/8 restricted	None known
Specific disease marker	Autoantibodies to TG2	Not yet identified	For the majority: not yet identified	none
Enteropathy Inflammation	Moderate-severe	Mild, "unspecific" (increased IEL)	Mild, "unspecific" (IEL, eosinophils)	none
Symptoms (prevalence)	Intestinal and extra-intestinal (1%)	Intestinal and **extra-intestinal** (5-10%)	Intestinal and extra-intestinal (3-4%)	Intestinal (bloa-ting, diarrhea)
Complications	Co-morbidities and long term complications	Co-morbidities and long term complications	Short-and long-term complications (anaphylaxis; **IBS**)	None (rather: beneficial for gut health)

ATI amylase trypsin inhibitor(s), *FODMAPs* fermentable oligo-, di-, monosaccharides and polyols (certain carbohydrates from plants); *HLA DQ2/8*—human lymphocyte antigen (major genetic predisposition for celiac disease, present in all patients), *IBS* irritable bowel syndrome

Selected Key References with Comments

Introduction

Lieberman S (2006). The Gluten Connection: How Gluten Sensitivity May Be Sabotaging Your Health - And What You Can Do to Take Control Now. Rodale, Emmaus, PA.

Davis W (2012). Wheat Belly. HarperCollins, New York, NY.

Perlmutter D (2013). Brain Grain: The Surprising Truth about Wheat, Carbs, and Sugar -Your Brain's Silent Killers. Little, Brown and Company, Columbus, GA.

Osborne P (2016). No Grain – no Pain. A 30-Day Diet for Eliminating the Root Cause of Chronic Pain. Simon and Schuster, New York, NY.

→ Popular books focused on gluten, with partly nonscientific or unfounded hypotheses and allegations. None of the authors is a renowned expert scientist or clinician in the field of wheat and wheat related diseases.

Fasano A (2014). Gluten Freedom. John Wiley and Sons, Hoboken, NJ.

→ Popular science book with a narrative aspect.

Schuppan D und Gisbert-Schuppan K (2018). Tägliches Brot: Krank durch Weizen, Gluten und ATI. Springer Medizin, Heidelberg, Germany.

→ The first book on the 3 mechanistically and clinically defined, inflammatory wheat sensitivities (in German). The precursor of the present book on the wheat syndromes.

© Springer Nature Switzerland AG 2019

D. Schuppan, K. Gisbert-Schuppan, *Wheat Syndromes*

https://doi.org/10.1007/978-3-030-19023-1

Wheat, gluten, ATI: an overview

Bonjean AP, Angus WJ (2001). The World Wheat Book: A History of Wheat. Cachan, Lavoisier.

→ Thorough overview of the history, cultivation, breeding and processing of wheat.

Tanno K, Willcox G. How fast was wild wheat domesticated? *Science* 2006;311:1886.
Kislev ME, Weiss E, Hartmann A. Impetus for sowing and the beginning of agriculture: ground collecting of wild cereals. *Proc Natl Acad Sci U S A* 2004;101:2692-5.

→ Overview of grains, wild wheats up to their systematic cultivation.

Charmet G. Wheat domestication: lessons for the future. C R Biol 2011;334:212-20.

→ Wheat breeding, from the ancient diploid to the modern hexaploid wheat.

International Wheat Genome Sequencing Consortium (IWGSC, more than 200 authors). Shifting the limits in wheat research and breeding using a fully annotated reference genome. *Science* 2018; 361(6403);eaar7191.
Ramírez-González RH, Borrill P, Lang D, Harrington SA, Brinton J, Venturini L, Davey M, Jacobs J, van Ex F, Pasha A, Khedikar Y, Robinson SJ, Cory AT, Florio T, Concia L, Juery C, Schoonbeek H, Steuernagel B, Xiang D, Ridout CJ, Chalhoub B, Mayer KFX, Benhamed M, Latrasse D, Bendahmane A; International Wheat Genome Sequencing Consortium, Wulff BBH, Appels R, Tiwari V, Datla R, Choulet F, Pozniak CJ, Provart NJ, Sharpe AG, Paux E, Spannagl M, Bräutigam A, Uauy C. The transcriptional landscape of polyploid wheat. *Science* 2018;361(6403);eaar6089
Brenchley R, Spannagl M, Pfeifer M, Barker GL, D'Amore R, Allen AM, McKenzie N, Kramer M, Kerhornou A, Bolser D, Kay S, Waite D, Trick M, Bancroft I, Gu Y, Huo N, Luo MC, Sehgal S, Gill B, Kianian S, Anderson O, Kersey P, Dvorak J, McCombie WR, Hall A, Mayer KF, Edwards KJ, Bevan MW, Hall N. Analysis of the bread wheat genome using whole-genome shotgun sequencing. *Nature* 2012;29;491:705-10.

→ The complete genome and transcriptome of modern hexaploid bread wheat has been decoded; it contains 94,000-96,000 genes, i.e., roughly four times as many as the human genome.

Juhász A, Belova T, Florides CG, Maulis C, Fischer I, Gell G, Birinyi Z, Ong J, Keeble-Gagnère G, Maharajan A, Ma W, Gibson P, Jia J, Lang D, Mayer KFX, Spannagl M; International Wheat Genome Sequencing Consortium, Tye-Din JA,

Appels R, Olsen OA. Genome mapping of seed-borne allergens and immunoresponsive proteins in wheat. *Sci Adv* 2018;4:eaar8602.

Guo G, Lv D, Yan X, et al. Proteome characterization of developing grains in bread wheat cultivars (Triticum aestivum L.). *BMC Plant Biol* 2012;12:147.

Nadolska-Orczyk A, Rajchel IK, Orczyk W, Gasparis S. Major genes determining yield-related traits in wheat and barley. *Theor Appl Genet* 2017;130:1081-98.

> → Relevant advances in describing and charting functionally relevant wheat proteins.

Wieser H. Chemistry of gluten proteins. *Food Microbiol* 2007;24:115-9.

> → Overview on the multitude of different gluten proteins and their chemical properties.

Dupont FM, Vensel WH, Tanaka CK, Hurkman WJ, Altenbach SB. Deciphering the complexities of the wheat flour proteome using quantitative two-dimensional electrophoresis, three proteases and tandem mass spectrometry. *Proteome Sci* 2011;9:10.

> → Quantitative Analysis of a modern bread wheat with a special focus on ATI.

Schuppan D, Zevallos V. Wheat amylase trypsin inhibitors as nutritional activators of innate immunity. *Dig Dis* 2015;33:260–3.

> → First overview on the pro-inflammatory role of wheat ATI.

Immunology of the intestine

MacDonald TT, Monteleone I, Fantini MC, Monteleone G. Regulation of homeostasis and inflammation in the intestine. *Gastroenterology* 2011;140:1768-75

Abraham C, Medzhitov R. Interactions between the host innate immune system and microbes in inflammatory bowel disease. *Gastroenterology* 2011;140:1729-37.

Bain CC, Mowat AM. Macrophages in intestinal homeostasis and inflammation. *Immunol Rev* 2014;260:102-17.

Postler TS, Ghosh S. Understanding the Holobiont: How microbial metabolites affect human health and shape the immune system. *Cell Metab.* 2017;26:110-130.

Honda K, Littman DR. The microbiota in adaptive immune homeostasis and disease. *Nature.* 2016;535:75-84.

> → Overviews on the immunology of the gut: the role of macrophages and the intestinal microbiome.

Powell N, Walker MM, Talley NJ. The mucosal immune system: master regulator of bidirectional gut-brain communications. *Nat Rev Gastroenterol Hepatol* 2017;14:143-159.

> → Review of how the intestinal microbiome affects the central nervous system.

González-Castro AM, Martínez C, Salvo-Romero E, Fortea M, Pardo-Camacho C, Pérez-Berezo T, Alonso-Cotoner C, Santos J, Vicario M. Mucosal pathobiology and molecular signature of epithelial barrier dysfunction in the small intestine in irritable bowel syndrome. *J Gastroenterol Hepatol* 2017;32:53-63.

> → Review of the causes of an increased intestinal permeability, i.e., the "leaky gut", demonstrating that gut leakiness is rather the consequence than the precondition for intestinal inflammation. Nonetheless, an increased leakiness can further promote inflammation, closing a vicious circle.

Pinto-Sanchez MI, Hall GB, Ghajar K, Nardelli A, Bolino C, Lau JT, Martin FP, Cominetti O, Welsh C, Rieder A, Traynor J, Gregory C, De Palma G, Pigrau M, Ford AC, Macri J, Berger B, Bergonzelli G, Surette MG, Collins SM, Moayyedi P, Bercik P. Probiotic Bifidobacterium longum NCC3001 Reduces Depression Scores and Alters Brain Activity: A Pilot Study in Patients With Irritable Bowel Syndrome. *Gastroenterology* 2017;153:448-459.

> → The first clinical study showing that beneficial (probiotic) bacteria taken on a regular basis improve symptoms of depression, confirming the gut-brain axis not only for classical inflammatory CNS diseases like multiple sclerosis, but also for CNS diseases that were believed to be largely non-inflammatory.

Celiac disease and its manifold manifestations

Catassi C, Fabiani E, Rätsch IM, Coppa GV, Giorgi PL, Pierdomenico R, Alessandrini S, Iwanejko G, Domenici R, Mei E, Miano A, Marani M, Bottaro G, Spina M, Dotti M, Montanelli A, Barbato M, Viola F, Lazzari R, Vallini M, Guariso G, Plebani M, Cataldo F, Traverso G, Ventura A, et al. The coeliac ice-berg in Italy. A multicentre antigliadin antibodies screening for coeliac disease in school-age subjects. *Acta Paediatr Suppl* 1996;412:29-35.

> → First report of the high prevalence (disease occurrence) of celiac disease in Italy as detected by screening for celiac autoantibodies EMA) and confirmation by endoscopy and duodenal biopsies in school children, most of whom had few or atypical symptoms (the celiac iceberg).

Lionetti E, Gatti S, Pulvirenti A, Catassi C. Celiac disease from a global perspective. *Best Pract Res Clin Gastroenterol* 2015;29:365-79.

→ Overview of the worldwide prevalence of celiac disease.

Lundin KE, Scott H, Hansen T, Paulsen G, Halstensen TS, Fausa O, Thorsby E, Sollid LM. Gliadin-specific, HLA-DQ(alpha 1∗0501,beta 1∗0201) restricted T cells isolated from the small intestinal mucosa of celiac disease patients. *J Exp Med* 1993;178:187-96.

Lundin KE, Sollid LM, Qvigstad E, Markussen G, Gjertsen HA, Ek J, Thorsby E. T lymphocyte recognition of a celiac disease-associated cis- or trans-encoded HLA-DQ alpha/beta-heterodimer. *J Immunol* 1990;145:136-9.

→ First description of the primary genetic predisposition (HLA-DQ2) for celiac disease and its role in intestinal T cell activation.

Dieterich W, Ehnis T, Bauer M, Donner P, Volta U, Riecken EO, Schuppan D. Identification of tissue transglutaminase as the autoantigen of celiac disease. *Nat Med* 1997;3:797-801.

→ Discovery and characterization of tissue transglutaminase (TG2) as celiac disease autoantigen.

Dieterich W, Laag E, Schöpper H, Volta U, Ferguson A, Gillett H, Riecken EO, Schuppan D. Autoantibodies to tissue transglutaminase as predictors of celiac disease. *Gastroenterology* 1998;115:1317-21.

Sulkanen S, Halttunen T, Laurila K, Kolho KL, Korponay-Szabó IR, Sarnesto A, Savilahti E, Collin P, Mäki M. Tissue transglutaminase autoantibody enzyme-linked immunosorbent assay in detecting celiac disease. *Gastroenterology* 1998;115:1322-8.

→ First description of the blood test to detect celiac disease, now in use worldwide, based on IgA antibodies to TG2.

Molberg O, Mcadam SN, Körner R, Quarsten H, Kristiansen C, Madsen L, Fugger L, Scott H, Norén O, Roepstorff P, Lundin KE, Sjöström H, Sollid LM. Tissue transglutaminase selectively modifies gliadin peptides that are recognized by gut-derived T cells in celiac disease. *Nat Med* 1998;4:713-7.

van de Wal Y, Kooy Y, van Veelen P, Peña S, Mearin L, Papadopoulos G, Koning F. Selective deamidation by tissue transglutaminase strongly enhances gliadin-specific T cell reactivity. *J Immunol* 1998;161:1585-8.

→ Elucidation of the exact mechanism by which the autoantigen and enzyme TG2 modifies gluten peptides via deamidation to make them better binders to HLA-DQ2 und HLA-DQ8, and therefore highly potent T cell activators.

Schuppan D, Junker Y, Barisani D. Celiac Disease: From Pathogenesis to novel therapies. *Gastroenterology* 2009;137:1912-33.

Kelly CP, Bai JC, Liu E, Leffler DA. Advances in diagnosis and management of celiac disease. *Gastroenterology* 2015;148:1175-86.

Lebwohl B, Sanders DS, Green PHR. Coeliac disease. *Lancet* 2018;391:70-81.

→ General reviews on the manifold aspects of celiac disease.

Rubio-Tapia A, Hill ID, Kelly CP, Calderwood AH, Murray JA; American College of Gastroenterology. ACG clinical guidelines: diagnosis and management of celiac disease. *Am J Gastroenterol* 2013 May;108(5):656-76.

→ US clinical guidelines for the diagnosis and management of celiac disease, including differential diagnoses.

Ludvigsson JF, Bai JC, Biagi F, Card TR, Ciacci C, Ciclitira PJ, Green PH, Hadjivassiliou M, Holdoway A, van Heel DA, Kaukinen K, Leffler DA, Leonard JN, Lundin KE, McGough N, Davidson M, Murray JA, Swift GL, Walker MM, Zingone F, Sanders DS; BSG Coeliac Disease Guidelines Development Group; British Society of Gastroenterology. Diagnosis and management of adult coeliac disease: guidelines from the British Society of Gastroenterology. *Gut* 2014 Aug;63(8):1210-28.

→ UK clinical guidelines for the diagnosis and management of celiac disease.

Felber J, Aust D, Baas S, Bischoff S, Bläker H, Daum S, Keller R, Koletzko S, Laass M, Nothacker M, Roeb E, Schuppan D, Stallmach A. [Results of a S2k-Consensus Conference of the German Society of Gastroenterology, Digestive- and Metabolic Diseases (DGVS) in conjunction with the German Coeliac Society (DZG)regarding coeliac disease, wheat allergy and wheat sensitivity]. *Z Gastroenterol* 2014;52:711-43.

→ German guidelines for the diagnosis and treatment of celiac disease, including the differential diagnoses wheat allergy and "non-celiac wheat sensitivity".

Bai JC, Fried M, Corazza GR, Schuppan D, Farthing M, Catassi C, Greco L, Cohen H, Ciacci C, Eliakim R, Fasano A, González A, Krabshuis JH, LeMair A. World gastroenterology organisation global guidelines on celiac disease. *J Clin Gastroenterol* 2013;47:121-6.

→ First global clinical guidelines on the management of celiac disease.

Jabri B, Sollid LM. T Cells in celiac disease. *J Immunol* 2017;198:3005-14.

→ Overview of the T cell immunology of celiac disease.

Vriezinga SL, Auricchio R, Bravi E, Castillejo G, Chmielewska A, Crespo Escobar P, Kolaček S, Koletzko S, Korponay-Szabo IR, Mummert E, Polanco I, Putter H,

Ribes-Koninckx C, Shamir R, Szajewska H, Werkstetter K, Greco L, Gyimesi J, Hartman C, Hogen Esch C, Hopman E, Ivarsson A, Koltai T, Koning F, Martinez-Ojinaga E, te Marvelde C, Pavic A, Romanos J, Stoopman E, Villanacci V, Wijmenga C, Troncone R, Mearin ML. Randomized feeding intervention in infants at high risk for celiac disease. *N Engl J Med* 2014;371:1304-15.

Lionetti E, Castellaneta S, Francavilla R, Pulvirenti A, Tonutti E, Amarri S, Barbato M, Barbera C, Barera G, Bellantoni A, Castellano E, Guariso G, Limongelli MG, Pellegrino S, Polloni C, Ughi C, Zuin G, Fasano A, Catassi C; SIGENP (Italian Society of Pediatric Gastroenterology, Hepatology, and Nutrition) Working Group on Weaning and CD Risk. Introduction of gluten, HLA status, and the risk of celiac disease in children. *N Engl J Med* 2014;371:1295-303.

→ The prospective study by Vriezinga et al. demonstrated that 4.5-5.9% of children with a risk to develop celiac disease (at least one parent with celiac disease and therefore the necessary disease genetic predisposition: HLA-DQ2 or HLA-DQ8) developed celiac disease at age 3. Unexpectedly, the careful introduction of low amounts of gluten between week 16 and 24 after birth, aimed at the induction of oral tolerance, did not reduce the emergence of celiac disease.

→ Lionetti et al. followed children with the same risk factors and found that feeding of substantial amounts of gluten at age 6 months vs 12 months led to an earlier manifestation of celiac disease at age 2. Thus, at age 5 the prevalence of celiac disease was comparable between both groups, reaching 16. Breastfeeding did reduce the number of children who developed celiac disease. The risk was increased twofold in carriers of 2 copies of the HLA-DQ2 gene compared to 1 copy.

Leffler DA, Schuppan D. Update on serologic testing in celiac disease. *Am J Gastroenterol* 2010;105:2520-4.

Husby S, Murray JA, Katzka DA. AGA Clinical practice update on diagnosis and monitoring of celiac disease: Changing utility of serology and histologic measures: Expert review. *Gastroenterology* 2019;156:885-9.

→ Review and guidelines on the serological diagnosis of celiac disease.

Ventura A, Magazzù G, Greco L. Duration of exposure to gluten and risk for auto-immune disorders in patients with celiac disease. SIGEP Study Group for Autoimmune Disorders in Celiac Disease. *Gastroenterology* 1999;117:297-303.

→ First report on the high prevalence (occurrence) of autoimmune diseases in patients with celiac disease, reaching around 30% when celiac disease is diagnosed in adulthood.

Leffler DA, Green PH, Fasano A. Extraintestinal manifestations of coeliac disease. *Nat Rev Gastroenterol Hepatol* 2015;12:561-71.

→ Extraintestinal manifestations of celiac disease.

Kahaly GJ, Frommer L, Schuppan D. Celiac disease and endocrine autoimmunity-the genetic link. *Autoimmun Rev* 2018;17:1169-1175.
Kahaly GJ, Frommer L, Schuppan D. Celiac disease and glandular autoimmunity. *Nutrients* 2018;10(7).
Verdu EF, Danska JS. Common ground: shared risk factors for type 1 diabetes and celiac disease. *Nat Immunol* 2018;19:685-695.
Lerner A, Wusterhausen P, Matthias T. Autoimmunity in celiac disease: Extra-intestinal manifestations. *Autoimmun Rev* 2019; 18:241-246.

→ Celiac disease and its association with endocrine and general autoimmunity.

van Gils T, Nijeboer P, van Wanrooij RL, Bouma G, Mulder CJ. Mechanisms and management of refractory coeliac disease. *Nat Rev Gastroenterol Hepatol* 2015;12:572-9.
Malamut G, Cellier C. Refractory celiac disease: epidemiology and clinical mani-festations. *Dig Dis* 2015;33:221-6.

→ Overviews of diagnosis and therapy of refractory celiac disease and intestinal T cell lymphoma.

Schuppan D, Junker Y, Barisani D. Celiac Disease: From Pathogenesis to novel therapies. *Gastroenterology* 2009;137:1912-33.
Mukherjee R, Kelly CP, Schuppan D. Nondietary therapies for celiac disease. *Gastrointest Endosc Clin N Am* 2012;22:811-31.
Kaukinen K, Lindfors K, Maki M. Advances in the treatment of coeliac disease: an immunopathogenic perspective. *Nat Rev Gastroenterol Hepatol* 2014;11:36-44.
Lundin KE, Sollid LM. Advances in coeliac disease. *Curr Opin Gastroenterol* 2014;30:154-62.
McCarville JL, Caminero A, Verdu EF. Pharmacological approaches in celiac dis-ease. *Curr Opin Pharmacol* 2015;25:7-12.

→ Reviews of drug therapies that are considered or in development to treat celiac disease.

Ludvigsson JF, Ciacci C, Green PH, Kaukinen K, Korponay-Szabo IR, Kurppa K, Murray JA, Lundin KEA, Maki MJ, Popp A, Reilly NR, Rodriguez-Herrera A, Sanders DS, Schuppan D, Sleet S, Taavela J, Voorhees K, Walker MM, Leffler DA. Outcome measures in coeliac disease trials: the Tampere recommendations. *Gut* 2018;67:1410-1424.

> → Review of objective parameters to measure efficacy of novel therapies for celiac disease.

Catassi C, Fabiani E, Iacono G, D'Agate C, Francavilla R, Biagi F, Volta U, Accomando S, Picarelli A, De Vitis I, Pianelli G, Gesuita R, Carle F, Mandolesi A, Bearzi I, Fasano A. A prospective, double-blind, placebo-controlled trial to establish a safe gluten threshold for patients with celiac disease. *Am J Clin Nutr* 2007;85:160-6.

> → Study showing that the tiny amount of 50 mg gluten daily (the equivalent of a small noodle) can elicit intestinal inflammation in celiac patients within 2 weeks.

Leffler D, Schuppan D, Pallav K, Najarian R, Goldsmith JD, Hansen J, Kabbani T, Dennis M, Kelly CP. Kinetics of the histological, serological and symptomatic responses to gluten challenge in adults with coeliac disease. *Gut* 2013;62:996-1004.

> → Gluten challenge study in patients with celiac disease in remission (without signs of inflammation under a gluten free diet). After 2 weeks of provocation with 5 or 7 g gluten per day (approximately one-third of the average daily ingestion) 75% of patients develop intestinal inflammation, as assessed by endoscopy and biopsy. After another 2 weeks (already off gluten), most patients have developed positive serum autoantibodies to tissue transglutaminase (TG2).

Leffler DA, Kelly CP, Green PH, Fedorak RN, DiMarino A, Perrow W, Rasmussen H, Wang C, Bercik P, Bachir NM, Murray JA. Larazotide acetate for persistent symptoms of celiac disease despite a gluten-free diet: a randomized controlled trial. *Gastroenterology* 2015;148:1311-9.

> → A study that used the oral pharmacological agent Larazotide on the assumption of a prominent "leaky gut" in celiac disease. Larazotide had been supposed to decrease gut leakiness. Here, paradoxically the lowest dose but not the higher doses improved the clinical symptoms of celiac patients who were challenged with a small amount of gluten, having made interpretation of the results difficult. Moreover, it is unclear if the drug, even if effective in decreasing the "leakiness" would be effective in ameliorating inflammation upon gluten ingestion. A histological assessment pre- and post-challenge was not performed, currently being the primary measure of a drug's efficacy in phase 2 clinical studies.

Tye-Din JA, Stewart JA, Dromey JA, Beissbarth T, van Heel DA, Tatham A, Henderson K, Mannering SI, Gianfrani C, Jewell DP, Hill AV, McCluskey J, Rossjohn J, Anderson RP. Comprehensive, quantitative mapping of T cell epitopes in gluten in celiac disease. *Sci Transl Med* 2010;2:41ra51.

> → Superb work defining 3 key (immuno-dominant) gluten peptides from wheat and barley as basis for a gluten vaccination aiming at inducing oral tolerance to gluten in celiac patients.

Lähdeaho ML, Kaukinen K, Laurila K, Vuotikka P, Koivurova OP, Kärjä-Lahdensuu T, Marcantonio A, Adelman DC, Mäki M. Glutenase ALV003 attenuates gluten-induced mucosal injury in patients with celiac disease. *Gastroenterology* 2014;146:1649-58.

> → First, well standardized pilot study showing that the oral ingestion of 2 gluten degrading enzymes (Latiglutenase) together with gluten-containing orange juice can suppress the otherwise gluten-induced inflammation in the small intestine.

Murray JA, Kelly CP, Green PH, Marcantonio A, Wu TT, Mäki M, Adelman DC; CeliAction Study Group of Investigators. No difference between Latiglutenase and placebo in reducing villous atrophy or improving symptoms in patients with symptomatic celiac disease. *Gastroenterology* 2017;152:787-798.

> → Real-life-follow-up study of 500 patients who had a moderately active celiac disease despite a gluten-free diet. Patients were treated either with Latiglutenase or placebo. This largest single drug study could not demonstrate a therapeutic effect of Latiglutenase, since both groups showed a moderate improvement. The improvement in the placebo patients (who did not receive active enzyme) was due to an improved compliance with the gluten-free diet under study conditions on the one hand, and to lower efficiency of the enzymes in a complex food mixture (in contrast to gluten that was suspended in a glass of orange juice in the above-mentioned study by Lähdeaho et al.).

Caminero A, Galipeau HJ, McCarville JL, Johnston CW, Bernier SP, Russell AK, Jury J, Herran AR, Casqueiro J, Tye-Din JA, Surette MG, Magarvey NA, Schuppan D, Verdu EF. Duodenal bacteria from patients with celiac disease and healthy subjects distinctly affect gluten breakdown and immunogenicity. *Gastroenterology* 2016;151:670-83.

> → First report that shows that defined bacteria from the small intestine and their enzymes need to work in combination (Lactobacilli, but also pseudomonas) to degrade immuno-genic gluten peptides.

Tian N, Wei G, Schuppan D, Helmerhorst EJ. Effect of Rothia mucilaginosa enzymes on gliadin (gluten) structure, deamidation, and immunogenic epitopes relevant to celiac disease. *Am J Physiol Gastrointest Liver Physiol* 2014;307:G769-76.

Wei G, Tian N, Siezen R, Schuppan D, Helmerhorst EJ. Identification of food-grade subtilisins as gluten-degrading enzymes to treat celiac disease. *Am J Physiol Gastrointest Liver Physiol* 2016;311:G571-80.

> → Isolation of novel, gluten degrading proteases from bacteria that normally colonize the oral cavity and/or the gut. These bacteria and enzymes may lead to novel enzyme therapies for celiac disease.

Wolf C, Siegel JB, Tinberg C, Camarca A, Gianfrani C, Paski S, Guan R, Montelione G, Baker D, Pultz IS. Engineering of Kuma030: A Gliadin Peptidase That Rapidly Degrades Immunogenic Gliadin Peptides in Gastric Conditions. *J Am Chem Soc* 2015;137:13106-13.

> → A synthetic enzyme that currently has the highest gluten degrading activity in vitro and in vivo. A clinical study is planned.

Goel G, King T, Daveson AJ, Andrews JM, Krishnarajah J, Krause R, Brown GJE, Fogel R, Barish CF, Epstein R, Kinney TP, Miner PB Jr, Tye-Din JA, Girardin A, Taavela J, Popp A, Sidney J, Mäki M, Goldstein KE, Griffin PH, Wang S, Dzuris JL, Williams LJ, Sette A, Xavier RJ, Sollid LM, Jabri B, Anderson RP. Epitope-specific immunotherapy targeting CD4-positive T cells in coeliac disease: two randomised, double-blind, placebo-controlled phase 1 studies. *Lancet Gastroenterol Hepatol* 2017;2:479-493.

> → First clinical data on the tolerability and safety of gluten vaccination to generate oral tolerance to ingested gluten in celiac patients. A placebo-controlled study to test its efficacy is planned.

Jamma S, Leffler DA, Dennis M, Najarian RM, Schuppan D, Sheth S, Kelly CP. Small intestinal release mesalamine for the treatment of refractory celiac disease type I. *J Clin Gastroenterol* 2011;45:30-3.

> → A small clinical study on the efficacy of 5-ASA, a mild anti-inflammatory drug that is used to maintain remission in patients with inflammatory bowel disease, to treat refractory celiac disease type 1.

Mukewar SS, Sharma A, Rubio-Tapia A, Wu TT, Jabri B, Murray JA. Open-Capsule Budesonide for Refractory Celiac Disease. Am J Gastroenterol 2017;112:959-967.

> → Study showing a high response rate of patients with a mild RDC type 2 to an oral corticosteroid.

ATI-sensitivity

Junker Y, Zeissig S, Kim SJ, Barisani D, Wieser H, Leffler DA, Zevallos V, Libermann TA, Dillon S, Freitag TL, Kelly CP, Schuppan D. Wheat amylase trypsin inhibitors drive intestinal inflammation via activation of toll-like receptor 4. *J Exp Med* 2012;209:2395-408.

> → First report on ATI as triggers of intestinal inflammation. Identification of TLR4 as ATI-receptor on macrophages and dendritic cells.

Oda Y, Matsunaga T, Fukuyama K, Miyazaki T, Morimoto T. Tertiary and quaternary structures of 0.19 alpha-amylase inhibitor from wheat kernel determined by X-ray analysis at 2.06 A resolution. *Biochemistry* 1997;36:13503-11.

> → First and currently the only X-ray structural analysis of a wheat ATI.

Altenbach SB, Vensel WH, Dupont FM. The spectrum of low molecular weight alpha-amylase/protease inhibitor genes expressed in the US bread wheat cultivar Butte 86. *BMC Res. Notes* 2011;4:242.

> → Exhaustive proteomic analysis of ATI in a modern bread wheat. 11 ATI species were detected amounting to about 3% of the wheat protein

Catassi C, Bai JC, Bonaz B, Bouma G, Calabrò A, Carroccio A, Castillejo G, Ciacci C, Cristofori F, Dolinsek J, Francavilla R, Elli L, Green P, Holtmeier W, Koehler P, Koletzko S, Meinhold C, Sanders D, Schumann M, Schuppan D, Ullrich R, Vécsei A, Volta U, Zevallos V, Sapone A, Fasano A. non-celiac gluten sensitivity: the new frontier of gluten related disorders. *Nutrients* 2013;5:3839-53.

Catassi C, Alaedini A, Bojarski C, Bonaz B, Bouma G, Carroccio A, Castillejo G, De Magistris L, Dieterich W, Di Liberto D, Elli L, Fasano A, Hadjivassiliou M, Kurien M, Lionetti E, Mulder CJ, Rostami K, Sapone A, Scherf K, Schuppan D, Trott N, Volta U, Zevallos V, Zopf Y, Sanders DS. The overlapping area of non-celiac gluten sensitivity (NCGS) and wheat-sensitive irritable bowel syndrome (IBS): An update. *Nutrients* 2017;9(11).

> → International consensus reports on "non-celiac gluten sensitivity" or correctly: "non-celiac wheat sensitivity". Awareness of ATI as a plausible cause of mainly extra-intestinal manifestations and the connection of intestinal manifestations with IBS.

Schuppan D, Zevallos V. Wheat amylase trypsin inhibitors as nutritional activators of innate immunity. *Dig Dis* 2015;33:260-3.

Fasano A, Sapone A, Zevallos V, Schuppan D. Non-celiac Gluten Sensitivity. *Gastroenterology* 2015;148:1195-204.

Schuppan D, Pickert G, Ashfaq-Khan M, Zevallos V. Non-celiac wheat sensitivity: differential diagnosis, triggers and implications. *Best Pract Res Clin Gastroenterol* 2015;29:469-76.

> → Reviews on the pro-inflammatory effects of ATI.

Cuccioloni M, Mozzicafreddo M, Bonfili L, Cecarini V, Giangrossi M, Falconi M, Saitoh SI, Eleuteri AM, Angeletti M. Interfering with the high-affinity interaction between wheat amylase trypsin inhibitor CM3 and toll-like receptor 4: in silico and biosensor-based studies. *Sci Rep* 2017;7:13169.

> → Identification of a peptide sequence in ATI CMR that mediates interaction with TLR4.

Zevallos VF, Raker V, Tenzer S, Jimenez-Calvente C, Ashfaq-Khan M, Rüssel N, Pickert G, Schild H, Steinbrink K, Schuppan D. Nutritional wheat amylase-trypsin inhibitors promote intestinal inflammation via activation of myeloid cells. *Gastroenterology* 2017;152:1100-1113.

> → This research report shows for the first time that nutritional ATI worsen pre-existing intestinal inflammation in experimental inflammatory bowel disease. It also suggests that, once activated by ATI, intestinal dendritic cells appear to leave the gut mucosa towards the surrounding mesenteric lymph nodes and possibly further into peripheral organs. ATI in the food also induce a marked systemic inflammatory response, as can be measured by blood cytokine and chemokine elevations.

Zevallos VF, Raker VK, Maxeiner J, Scholtes P, Steinbrink K, Schuppan D. Dietary wheat amylase trypsin inhibitors exacerbate murine allergic airway inflammation. *Eur J Clin Nutr* 2018;58:1507-14.

Bellinghausen I, Weigmann B, Zevallos V, Maxeiner J, Reissig S, Waisman A, Schuppan D, Saloga J. Wheat amylase/trypsin inhibitors exacerbate intestinal and airway allergic immune responses in humanized mice. *J Allergy Clin Immunol* 2019;143:201-212.e4.

> → First reports on the promotion of respiratory and food allergies by nutritional ATI. In the second study, mice were studies that had a "humanized immune system". Here, most of the murine immune cells were replaced by immune cells of allergic patients compared to healthy controls. ATI promoted allergies against a broad range of common allergens.

Pickert G, Wirtz S, Heck R, Rosigkeit S, Thies D, Ashfaq-Khan M, Surabattula R, Ehmann D, Wehkamp J, Aslam M, He GW, Weigert A, Foerster F, Becker C, Bockamp E, Schuppan D. Wheat consumption aggravates experimental colitis by amylase trypsin inhibitor (ATI)-mediated dysbiosis. *Gastroenterology* 2019, in press.

Caminero A, McCarville JL, Zevallos VF, Pigrau M, Yu XB, Jury J, Galipeau HJ, Clarizio AV, Casqueiro J, Murray JA, Collins SM, Alaedini A, Bercik P, Schuppan D, Verdu EF. Lactobacilli degrade wheat amylase trypsin inhibitors (ATI) and ameliorate gut dysfunction induced by immunogenic wheat proteins. *Gastroenterology* 2019;156:2266-2280.

> → These 2 studies show that, apart from activating TLR4, ATI have 2 additional activities that explain their potent disease-promoting effect: 1. ATI directly cause intestinal dysbiosis and worsen pre-existing gut inflammation by acting as a selective antibiotic for certain beneficial intestinal bacteria; transplantation of ATI-conditioned stool into mice promotes their colitis. 2. ATI induce "a leaky gut", i.e. increase intestinal permeability and thus favor inflammation; certain lactobacilli can partly degrade ATI; this may lead to the development of probiotics that reduce ATI concentrations in the intestine.

Ashfaq-Khan M, Aslam M, Qureshi MA, Senkowski MS, Weng SY, Strand D, Kim YO, Schattenberg, JM, Schuppan D. Dietary wheat amylase trypsin inhibitors promote obesity and non-alcoholic fatty liver disease. *Gut* 2019, in revision.

> → ATI consumption promotes weight gain, type 2 diabetes, adipose tissue inflammation, fatty liver disease and liver fibrosis in mice on a hyper-caloric, high fat diet; the weight gain compared to mice fed the same diet without ATI is due to a change in the gut microbiota that increases the energy harvest form the consumed food, despite equal amounts of consumed food.

Uhde M, Ajamian M, Caio G, De Giorgio R, Indart A, Green PH, Verna EC, Volta U, Alaedini A. Intestinal cell damage and systemic immune activation in individuals reporting sensitivity to wheat in the absence of coeliac disease. *Gut* 2016;65:1930-1937.

> → This study identified several blood markers of (innate) immune activation that are elevated in many patients with "non-celiac wheat sensitivity" compared to healthy controls. Most patients displayed symptoms either of atypical wheat allergy or ATI-sensitivity. The results confirm the inflammatory nature of the wheat sensitivities.

Laktose-, fructose- und histamin intolerance: overdiagnosed and overrated

San Mauro Martin I, Brachero S, Garicano Vilar E. Histamine intolerance and dietary management: A complete review. Allergol Immunopathol (Madr) 2016;44:475-83.

Maintz L, Novak N. Histamine and histamine intolerance. *Am J Clin Nutr* 2007;85:1185-96.

→ Reviews on histamine intolerance that is still considered an ill-defined condition in most cases.

Turnbull JL, Adams HN, Gorard DA. Review article: the diagnosis and management of food allergy and food intolerances. *Aliment Pharmacol Ther* 2015;41:3-25.

→ General review on classical food allergies and food intolerances.

Hammer HF, Hammer J. Diarrhea caused by carbohydrate malabsorption. *Gastroenterol Clin North Am* 2012;41:611-27.

→ Overview of lactose and fructose intolerance.

Schumann D, Klose P, Lauche R, Dobos G, Langhorst J, Cramer H. Low fermentable, oligo-, di-, mono-saccharides and polyol diet in the treatment of irritable bowel syndrome: A systematic review and meta-analysis. *Nutrition* 2018;45:24-31.

→ Meta-analysis of 9 reliable clinical studies subjecting patients with "irritable bowel syndrome" to a low FODMAP diet all short-term studies, lasting only for a few weeks, showing some efficacy in improving abdominal symptoms, but also a reduction of bacterial mass and potentially beneficial bacteria like Akkermansia and Bifidobacteria.

Catassi G, Lionetti E, Gatti S, Catassi C. The Low FODMAP Diet: Many Question Marks for a Catchy Acronym. *Nutrients* 2017;9.

→ Critical review on the clinical relevance of the FODMAP intolerance in patients with chronic intestinal complaints and on possible health risks of low FODMAP diets.

Classical and atypical food allergies - irritable bowel syndrome

Valenta R, Hochwallner H, Linhart B, Pahr S. Food allergies: the basics. *Gastroenterology* 2015;148:1120-31.

→ Review on all aspects of IgE-positive (classical) food allergies.

Salcedo G, Quirce S, az-Perales A. Wheat allergens associated with Baker's asthma. *J Investig Allergol Clin Immunol* 2011;21:81-92.

→ Report on wheat allergy and the multitude of wheat allergens in Baker's asthma.

Stapel SO, Asero R, Ballmer-Weber BK, Knol EF, Strobel S, Vieths S, Kleine-Tebbe J; EAACI Task Force. Testing for IgG4 against foods is not recommended as a diagnostic tool: EAACI Task Force Report. *Allergy* 2008;63:793-6.

→ European consensus guidelines discarding IgG allergen tests for the diagnosis of food allergies.

Fritscher-Ravens A, <u>Schuppan</u> D, Ellrichmann M, Schoch S, Röcken C, Brasch J, Bethge J, Böttner M, Klose J, Milla PJ. Confocal endomicroscopy shows food-associated changes in the intestinal mucosa of patients with irritable bowel syndrome. *Gastroenterology* 2014;147:1012-20.

→ The first report indicating that up to 70% of patients with the diagnosis of irritable bowel syndrome (IBS) have indeed an atypical food allergy. Subjects did not have IgE antibodies or a positive skin test reaction to the causative food, i.e. markers of classical allergies. Patients were sequentially challenged with 4 major suspected allergens: wheat, milk, soy and yeast. The Allergen solutions/suspensions were sequentially, every 5 minutes, sprayed onto the duodenal mucosa via the magnification endoscope (confocal laser endomicroscopy). In case of an atypical allergy, an immediate reaction, prominently extrusion of plasma fluid into the gut lumen, mucosal inflammatory cell infiltration and edema could be observed. These intestinal mucosal reactions occurred with 5 minutes, while abdominal symptoms developed up to several hours later. Wheat was the responsible allergen in more than half of the patients, and dietary exclusion of the identified allergen led to cure.

Fritscher-Ravens A, Pflaum T, Mösinger M, Ruchai Z, Röcken C, Milla PJ, Das M, Böttner M, Wedel T, <u>Schuppan</u> D. Many patients with irritable bowel syndrome have atypical food allergies not associated with IgE. *Gastroenterology* 2019;157:109-18.

→ This second report on atypical food allergies confirmed the results of the first report in a 3-fold higher number of patients. Wheat was responsible for the allergy and symptoms in 60% of the subjects. Analysis on the intestinal biopsies before and after positive food challenge demonstrated increased inflammatory cells, intraepithelial lymphocytes and eosinophil activation in the intestinal mucosa. Moreover, the allergens disturbed tight junctional integrity of the intestinal epithelium.

Index

© Springer Nature Switzerland AG 2019
D. Schuppan, K. Gisbert-Schuppan, *Wheat Syndromes*
https://doi.org/10.1007/978-3-030-19023-1